Lecture Notes of the Institute
for Computer Sciences, Social Informatics
and Telecommunications Engineering   530

Editorial Board Members

Ozgur Akan, *Middle East Technical University, Ankara, Türkiye*
Paolo Bellavista, *University of Bologna, Bologna, Italy*
Jiannong Cao, *Hong Kong Polytechnic University, Hong Kong, Hong Kong*
Geoffrey Coulson, *Lancaster University, Lancaster, UK*
Falko Dressler, *University of Erlangen, Erlangen, Germany*
Domenico Ferrari, *Università Cattolica Piacenza, Piacenza, Italy*
Mario Gerla, *UCLA, Los Angeles, USA*
Hisashi Kobayashi, *Princeton University, Princeton, USA*
Sergio Palazzo, *University of Catania, Catania, Italy*
Sartaj Sahni, *University of Florida, Gainesville, USA*
Xuemin Shen, *University of Waterloo, Waterloo, Canada*
Mircea Stan, *University of Virginia, Charlottesville, USA*
Xiaohua Jia, *City University of Hong Kong, Kowloon, Hong Kong*
Albert Y. Zomaya, *University of Sydney, Sydney, Australia*

The LNICST series publishes ICST's conferences, symposia and workshops.

LNICST reports state-of-the-art results in areas related to the scope of the Institute. The type of material published includes

- Proceedings (published in time for the respective event)
- Other edited monographs (such as project reports or invited volumes)

LNICST topics span the following areas:

- General Computer Science
- E-Economy
- E-Medicine
- Knowledge Management
- Multimedia
- Operations, Management and Policy
- Social Informatics
- Systems

Venere Ferraro · Mario Covarrubias ·
Eftim Zdravevski · Ivan Miguel Pires ·
José Manuel Marques Martins de Almeida ·
Norberto Jorge Gonçalves
Editors

IoT Technologies and Wearables for HealthCare

10th EAI International Conference, HealthyIoT 2023, and
4th EAI International Conference, HealthWear 2023
Bratislava, Slovakia, October 24–26, 2023
Proceedings

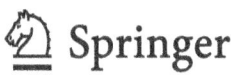

Editors
Venere Ferraro
Politecnico di Milano
Milan, Italy

Mario Covarrubias
Politecnico di Milano
Milan, Italy

Eftim Zdravevski
Ss. Cyril and Methodius University of Skopje
Skopje, North Macedonia

Ivan Miguel Pires
Universidade de Aveiro
Águeda, Portugal

José Manuel Marques Martins de Almeida
University of Trás-os-Montes e Alto Douro
Vila Real, Portugal

Norberto Jorge Gonçalves
University of Trás-os-Montes e Alto Douro
Vila Real, Portugal

ISSN 1867-8211　　　　　　　ISSN 1867-822X　(electronic)
Lecture Notes of the Institute for Computer Sciences, Social Informatics
and Telecommunications Engineering
ISBN 978-3-031-71910-3　　　ISBN 978-3-031-71911-0　(eBook)
https://doi.org/10.1007/978-3-031-71911-0

© ICST Institute for Computer Sciences, Social Informatics and Telecommunications Engineering 2024

This work is subject to copyright. All rights are solely and exclusively licensed by the Publisher, whether the whole or part of the material is concerned, specifically the rights of translation, reprinting, reuse of illustrations, recitation, broadcasting, reproduction on microfilms or in any other physical way, and transmission or information storage and retrieval, electronic adaptation, computer software, or by similar or dissimilar methodology now known or hereafter developed.
The use of general descriptive names, registered names, trademarks, service marks, etc. in this publication does not imply, even in the absence of a specific statement, that such names are exempt from the relevant protective laws and regulations and therefore free for general use.
The publisher, the authors and the editors are safe to assume that the advice and information in this book are believed to be true and accurate at the date of publication. Neither the publisher nor the authors or the editors give a warranty, expressed or implied, with respect to the material contained herein or for any errors or omissions that may have been made. The publisher remains neutral with regard to jurisdictional claims in published maps and institutional affiliations.

This Springer imprint is published by the registered company Springer Nature Switzerland AG
The registered company address is: Gewerbestrasse 11, 6330 Cham, Switzerland

If disposing of this product, please recycle the paper.

Preface

We are delighted to introduce the joint proceedings of the tenth edition of the European Alliance for Innovation (EAI) International Conference on IoT Technologies for HealthCare (HealthyIoT 2023) and the fourth edition of the European Alliance for Innovation (EAI) International Conference on Wearables in Healthcare (HealthWear 2023). Traditionally, the HealthyIoT conference covers multiple aspects of using IoT in healthcare and brings together technology experts, researchers, industry experts, and international authorities contributing to designing, developing, and deploying healthcare solutions based on IoT technologies, standards, and procedures. This year the emphasis was on using IoT in healthcare for societal benefit – towards improved health and wellbeing for everyone. The Healthwear conference began in 2016 in Budapest to bring together researchers, developers, and industry professionals to discuss the key issues of personal health data research, and has strengthened its focus on wearable devices and systems. The combination of wearable devices and personalized medicine is transforming the way we approach prevention, cure, and rehabilitation and enabling individuals to take charge of their health whilst providing healthcare providers with more data-driven insights to deliver targeted and effective treatments.

As the conferences both took place in Bratislava on the same dates, with such closely related topics, an alliance seemed perfect for this year's edition. The technical program of HealthyIoT 2023 consisted of 5 full papers, in oral presentation sessions at the conference. The oral sessions included high-quality technical presentations of the papers submitted to the HealthyIoT 2023 tracks. HealthWear 2023 also consisted of 5 major papers within the area of Wearables in Healthcare, with a focus both on user empowerment and the role of big data in navigating health realms.

Coordination with the steering chair, Imrich Chlamtac, was essential for the conferences' success. We sincerely appreciate his constant support and guidance. It was also a great pleasure to work with such an excellent organizing committee team for their hard work organizing and supporting the conference. In particular, the Technical Program Committee, led respectively by our HealthyIoT TPC Co-Chairs, Petre Lameski and Hugo Paredes, and our HealthWear TPC Chairs, Venere Ferraro and Mario Covarrubbias, coordinated and contributed to the peer-review process of technical papers, and made high-quality technical programs. We are also grateful to the Conference Managers, Kristina Havlickova and Patricia Gabajova, for their support, and to all the authors who submitted their papers to the HealthyIoT 2023 conference, sharing their knowledge, experience, and genuine enthusiasm.

We strongly believe that the HealthyIoT conference provides a good forum for all researchers, developers, and practitioners to discuss scientific and technical aspects that are relevant to IoT technologies for healthcare, with HealthWear a perfect forum for healthcare wearables. We expect future conferences to be as successful and stimulating as indicated by the contributions presented in this volume.

Norberto Jorge Gonçalves
Ivan Miguel Pires
Eftim Zdravevski
José Manuel Marques Martins de Almeida
João Pavão
Paolo Perego
Nicola Francesco Lopomo
Venere Ferraro
Mario Covarrubias

Organization

Steering Committee

Imrich Chlamtac — University of Trento, Italy

Organizing Committee (HealthyIoT)

General Chair

Norberto Jorge Gonçalves — University of Trás-os-Montes e Alto Douro, Portugal

General Co-chair

Ivan Miguel Pires — University of Aveiro, Portugal

Program Chairs

Eftim Zdravevski — Ss. Cyril and Methodius University in Skopje, North Macedonia
Daniel Moreira Alexandre — University of Trás-os-Montes e Alto Douro, Portugal
João Pavão — University of Trás-os-Montes e Alto Douro, Portugal

TPC Chairs and Co-chairs

Petre Lameski — Ss. Cyril and Methodius University in Skopje, North Macedonia
Hugo Paredes — University of Trás-os-Montes e Alto Douro, Portugal

Sponsorship and Exhibit Chair

Paulo Coelho — Polytechnic of Leiria, Portugal

Local Chair

António Gouveia — University of Trás-os-Montes e Alto Douro, Portugal

Workshops Chair

Rute Bastardo — University of Trás-os-Montes e Alto Douro, Portugal

Publicity and Social Media Chairs

Malik Amraoui — University of Trás-os-Montes e Alto Douro, Portugal
Francisco Marinho — University of Trás-os-Montes e Alto Douro, Portugal

Publications Chair

José Manuel M. M. de Almeida — University of Trás-os-Montes e Alto Douro, Portugal

Web Chair

Paulo Neves — Polytechnic Institute of Castelo Branco, Portugal

Posters and PhD Track Chair

Maria Adelaide Andrade — University of Trás-os-Montes e Alto Douro, Portugal

Panels Chair

Nuno M. Garcia — University of Lisbon, Portugal

Demos Chair

Marco Duarte Naia — University of Trás-os-Montes e Alto Douro, Portugal

Tutorials Chair

José Paulo Lousado Polytechnic Institute of Viseu, Portugal

Technical Program Committee

Abdul Hannan	University of Engineering and Technology, Taxila, Pakistan
António Godinho	Polytechnic Institute of Coimbra, Portugal
Ciprian Dobre	University Politehnica of Bucharest, Romania
Constandinos Mavromoustakis	University of Nicosia, Cyprus
Dusan Kokur	Technical University of Kosice, Slovakia
Faisal Hussain	University of Engineering and Technology, Taxila, Pakistan
Francisco Garcia Encinas	University of Salamanca, Spain
Hanna Denysyuk	Universidade da Beira Interior, Portugal
Hugo Silva	Instituto de Telecomunicações, Portugal
Ivan Chorbev	Ss. Cyril and Methodius University in Skopje, North Macedonia
Juliana Sá	Centro Hospitalar Universitário do Porto, Portugal
Kuldar Taveter	Tallinn University, Estonia
Luis Augusto Silva	University of Salamanca, Spain
Mónica Costa	Instituto Politécnico de Castelo Branco, Portugal
Nuno Cruz Garcia	Universidade de Lisboa, Portugal
Paulo Simões	University of Coimbra, Portugal
Piotr Lasek	University of Rzeszów, Poland
Rossitza Goleva	New Bulgarian University, Bulgaria
Serge Autexier	German Research Centre for Artificial Intelligence (DFKI), Germany
Vasco Ponciano	Instituto Politécnico de Castelo Branco, Portugal
Vladimir Trajkovik	Ss. Cyril and Methodius University in Skopje, North Macedonia

Organizing Committee (HealthWear)

General Chairs

Paolo Perego Politecnico di Milano, Italy
Nicola Francesco Lopomo University of Brescia, Italy

TPC Chairs

Venere Ferraro	Politecnico di Milano, Italy
Mario Covarrubbias	Politecnico di Milano, Italy

Publications Chair

Emilia Scalona	University of Brescia, Italy

Technical Program Committee

Venere Ferraro	Politecnico di Milano, Italy
Paolo Perego	Politecnico di Milano, Italy
Nicola Francesco Lopomo	University of Brescia, Italy
Roberto Sironi	Politecnico di Milano, Italy
Carlo Emilio Standoli	Politecnico di Milano, Italy
Giorgio Buratti	Politecnico di Milano, Italy
Paolo Bellitti	University of Brescia, Italy
Jaime Oscar Casas Piedrafita	Universitat Politècnica de Catalunya, Spain
Gema Hornero Ocaña	Universitat Politècnica de Catalunya, Spain
Massimiliano Pau	University of Cagliari, Italy
Giacomo Borachi	Politecnico di Milano, Italy
Mario Covarrubias	Politecnico di Milano, Italy
Giuseppe Andreoni	Politecnico di Milano, Italy
Angelo Davalli	INAIL, Italy
Marianne Graves	Aarhus University, Denmark
Emilia Scalona	University of Brescia, Italy
Ezio Preatoni	University of Bath, UK

Contents

IoT Technologies for HealthCare

Test and Validation of an Internet of Things Platform for Remote
Monitoring of Pregnant Women 3
   *Jorge Miranda, Stefan Rahr Wagner, Magdalena Mazur-Milecka,
and Jacek Ruminski*

Transforming Diabetes Care: A Review of IoT-Based Mobile Health
Systems 14
   Fiza Ashfaq, Abdul Ahad, Mudassar Hussain, and Filipe Madeira

Investigating the Use of Utility Monitoring as a Means of Recognizing
Activities of Daily Living (ADLs) to Enable Independent Living Among
People Living with Dementia 33
   *Ciarán Nugent, Damon Berry, Jonathan Turner, Michael Wilson,
Ann Marron, Julie Doyle, and Dympna O'Sullivan*

Enhancing Transparency and Trustworthiness of Healthcare IoT Data
with AWS: A Proposed Model 44
   Zahra Ali, Abdul Ahad, Filipe Madeira, and Ibraheem Shayea

Guidelines to Develop an Art Therapy APP to Control the Children's State
Anxiety in Mexico 57
   Julieta Martínez, Marcela E. Buitrón, and Edwing A. Almeida

Wearables in Healthcare

Commercial and Research-Based Wearable Devices in Spinal Postural
Analysis: A Systematic Review 65
   Narges Pourshahrokhi, Yitong Sun, and Ali Asadipour

Role of Big Data, AI and Deep Learning in Medical Image Training
Models and Decision Support System Using I4.0 Technologies 84
   Kavita Bhatt and S. Mohan Kumar

Generating Breathing Patterns in Real-Time: Low-Latency Respiratory
Phase Tracking From 25 Hz PPG 97
   *Ian Karman, Yue Sun, Rahil Soroushmojdehi, Jose A. Silva,
and Mostafa 'Neo' Mohsenvand*

Navigating Health Applications Realms: Consent Challenges and User
Empowerment in European Law 117
   Petra Müllerová

The Application of Virtual Reality in Enhancing Medical Education:
Benefits, Challenges, and Outlook for the Future 131
   Seydou Golo Barro, Delwêndé Serge Lebian Wilfried Nikiema,
   Yves Kantagba, and Pascal Staccini

Author Index 139

IoT Technologies for HealthCare

Test and Validation of an Internet of Things Platform for Remote Monitoring of Pregnant Women

Jorge Miranda[1(✉)], Stefan Rahr Wagner[1], Magdalena Mazur-Milecka[2], and Jacek Ruminski[2]

[1] Department of Engineering, Aarhus University, Aarhus Centrum, Denmark
jmiranda@au.dk, sw@ece.au.dk
[2] Biomedical Engineering Department, Gdansk University of Technology, Gdansk, Poland
{magdalena.milecka,jacek.ruminski}@pg.edu.pl

Abstract. The WODIA project develops Internet of Things (IoT) tools for the screening and long-term monitoring of women suffering from preeclampsia, a non-communicable disease affecting women during pregnancy. This includes performing home monitoring using an internet of thing (IoT) gateway device along with blood pressure and other medico devices as well as activity trackers. It is important that the tools developed are valid and reliable for both clinical and home use. The integration of the devices, the infrastructure, and the server components have not previously been systematically validated and evaluated for reliability during prolonged usage. The aim of this study is to validate the functionality of the WODIA healthcare IoT system, with special focus on the web API. To assess it, a set of tests were defined, and a series of tools were developed to enable testing of the components of the system. With this methodology in place, it was possible to validate several aspects of the system, in an initial development stage.

Keywords: Internet of Things · Healthcare · Test · Clinical Evaluation

1 Introduction

Around half a million women die each year while giving birth [1]. The two non-communicable diseases preeclampsia and gestational hypertension are the cause of more than 70,000 mothers and half million infants dying each year. Infants who survive often experience long-term health problems: cerebral palsy, chronic lung disease, blindness, and hearing loss [2].

Once preeclampsia is diagnosed it cannot be cured by other means than by caesarean section. Recent studies have shown promising new diagnostic approaches using an extensive screening and monitoring battery of biomarkers combined with maternal phenotype and history categorization which are then classified into a risk model. Based on this model, medical treatment with antiplatelet agents has been found to be effective [3].

A study aimed at investigating the use of machine learning algorithms for the early prediction of preeclampsia was presented in [4]. Classification into the high- or low-risk group was made on synthetic data created on the basis of parameter distributions from studies on real patients. The study verified the quality of risk prediction based on various biomarkers, patient groups and for various models. It showed prediction accuracy for the best models of over 96%.

For this planned screening and monitoring a health IoT system is being developed as part of the WODIA project [5], which will use machine learning and deep learning techniques based on healthcare data collected in the clinic and the home setting using health IoT equipment. The WODIA system is an IoT distributed system, which is composed by the following subsystems as shown in Fig. 1:

1) **WODIA Web:** a cloud application which allows healthcare staff and patients to monitor it is the health status of the individual patients, specifically it can visualize the measurements performed, and it allows for the remote management of health interventions and actions. Besides a user interface, WODIA Web also has an application programming interface (API) which enables integration of devices and applications into the ecosystem, as well as a decision support engine.
2) **WODIA IoT Gateway:** is an embedded health gateway device, which enables communication between local medio, presence, and tracker devices with the cloud application and API. The gateway supports Wi-Fi, Bluetooth (BLE), ZigBee and 4G. The device is based on the CARIOT + ecosystem [6, 7]. However, any gateway system can be used, due to the reliance on open standards.
3) **Mobile device:** smartphone or tablet with applications which support the WODIA Web API, which enables the participants to perform or monitor their health status. Patients can either use their own devices or will receive a dedicated project device.
4) **Health devices:** also referred to as medico devices, which are devices deployed at the patient's home or at the healthcare facility, which enable the participants to perform health measurements. Such devices include blood pressure monitors or weight scales, which support the communication protocols Bluetooth, Wi-Fi or Zigbee. The Omron M7 Intelli IT was selected as the primary healthcare device for home monitoring because it supports Bluetooth, specifically the standard Bluetooth GATT blood pressure service and it is validated and certified for use in pregnant population [8].

WODIA totals four distinct phases of screening and monitoring during a pregnancy. During the first phase (around week 12 of the pregnancy) the woman will be screened at an outpatient clinic with a range of biomedical and biochemical tests. The results of these tests are run through a decision support algorithm, and women who are deemed to be in high risk for later developing preeclampsia are selected for home monitoring during the second phase. This is the home monitoring phase, which lasts around 8 weeks, from week 12 to week 20. During this period, any disease symptoms will not yet be visible, but there will be several additional biomarkers, including a tendency to a rise in blood pressure. Thus, during this home monitoring phase 2, the main use case for the WODIA system is for the participants to perform blood pressure measurements. They are expected to perform three blood pressure measurements in the morning and three in the afternoon. For that, a patient has a blood pressure device at home, plus a gateway. The interaction between these components is depicted in Fig. 2. They may

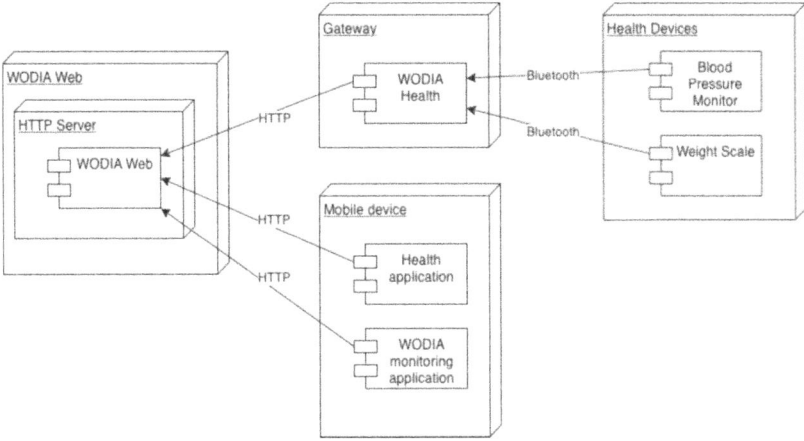

Fig. 1. UML Deployment diagram of the WODIA system architecture.

use their smartphone or a computer with a browser to review the results. It is important that measurements are performed at the same time and under the same circumstances to avoid bias in the measurements, which could affect the decision support algorithms.

Assuring high quality data implies assuring that not only the device, but the entire architecture performs reliably and valid. This implies that we need to test the architecture from device to API and to UI to ensure the entire system is valid and safe for clinical trials.

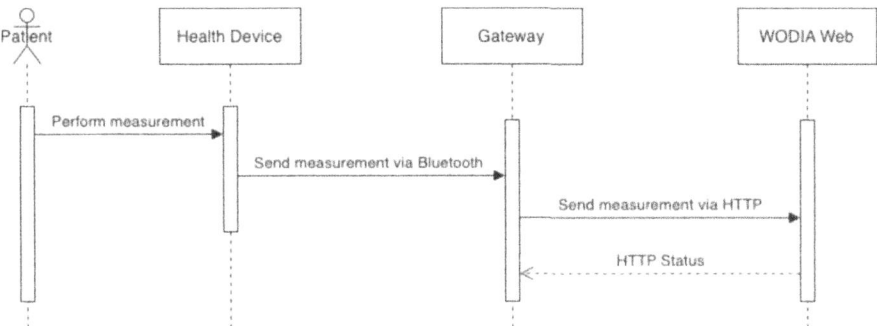

Fig. 2. UML Sequence diagram demonstrating how a blood pressure is performed by a patient in a home setting.

The Internet of Things has been a promising framework for enabling telemedicine applications, due to its distributed architecture and integration of heterogeneous network and computational technologies [9–12]. To meet the IoT goals of accuracy, interoperability, scalability, reliability, and security [9], thorough testing of an IoT system is needed. Although system testing is an established area, there are still open challenges on how to apply these techniques to IoT, mostly due to its cross-domain particularities present in its heterogenous and distributed nature [13–15]. Although some tools that try to address the challenges of testing IoT systems are available [13], research is required to understand how to better integrate this, because they generally focus in one part of the system (for example, testing embedded devices, or testing the cloud applications, or data processing), which makes assessing the state of the whole system difficult due to the numerous and heterogenous tools that exist [15].

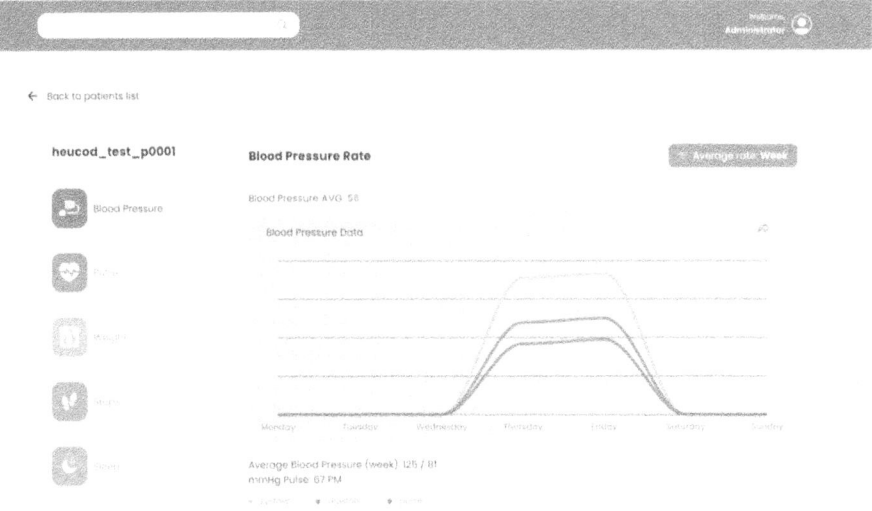

Fig. 3. Screenshot of the WODIA Web interface.

The aim of this study is to test and validate the functionality of the WODIA healthcare IoT system, with special focus on the web API, to enable faster integration of the multiple components of the system. This work gives contributions to the test methodologies in IoT systems and opens a discussion in the need to implement these methods in systems that generate clinical data, so that the quality of the datasets generated by these systems can be assured.

2 Methods

The integration of the gateways and mobile devices with the WODIA Web applications is made via the API. Therefore, to focus the assessment of the system, a series of acceptance and integration tests were initially defined. After, these were implemented using already existing testing tools (Tavern) it was also necessary to develop specific tools, specifically a patient's simulator and a UI tool to manage the Tavern tests.

Two acceptance tests were defined that will guide the whole testing effort:

- **AT1:** the API must implement CRUD (create-read-update-delete) HTTP requests for the device, device events, gateway, and user entities. Since all of them follow the CRUD pattern, each of the requests should comply with a standard set of success and error return codes (HTTP status code).

- **AT2:** the web platform must support multiple users sending events simultaneously and register all events.

The following strategies were implemented to assess the acceptance tests described above:

- for AT1 a black-box testing strategy was implemented, specifically integration tests were developed using the Tavern library (see Sect. 2.1) to test each of the endpoints of the API.
- for AT2, a custom simulator was developed in Python, that allows to simulate several users performing measurements in specific times of the day. This allows us to verify that the web application manages the data received correctly, and that it can run in the long term without any major issues. The interaction is made via the Web API tested in requirement 1.
- finally, still for AT2, a team outside the group that developed WODIA Web, performed manual testing with real blood pressure devices and visual assessment in the WODIA Web application UI, to verify that the performed measurements were successfully recorded and displayed.

Although other testing strategies such as unit tests, or module testing, were also used during the development of the system components, these are not within this publication's scope.

2.1 Integration Tests

As stated, a set of integration tests were defined, so that later they could be implemented in Tavern. In Table 1 the set of tests is described in a generic way, i.e. when implementing these tests, they will have to be implemented for each of the entities to test, specifically devices, device events, gateways and users.

Table 1. Table captions should be placed above the tables.

Test ID	Description	Expected HTTP status code
IT1	Successfully get all entities	200 OK
IT2	Successfully get existing entities, given an existing ID	200 OK
IT3	Fail to get a non-existing entity	404 Not found
IT4	Successfully create non-exiting entity	204 No content
IT5	Successfully create an entity with an ID with spaces	204 No content
IT6	Fail to create an entity whose request has an invalid payload (empty or missing fields)	400 Bad request
IT7	Fail to create repeated entities	400 Bad request
IT8	Fail to create entities whose ID fields are badly formed, such as empty string or NULL values	400 Bad request

(*continued*)

Table 1. (*continued*)

Test ID	Description	Expected HTTP status code
IT9	Successfully update an existing entity	204 No content
IT10	Fail to update a non-existing entity	404 Not found
IT11	Fail to update an entity whose request has an invalid payload (empty or missing fields)	400 Bad request
IT12	Successfully delete an existing entity	204 No content
IT13	Fail to delete a non-existing device	404 Not found
IT14	Fail to delete a non-specified device	400 Bad request
IT15	Successfully perform a request when the authentication token is set in the HTTP headers	200 OK or 204 No content
IT16	Fail to perform a request, because the authentication token in not sent in the HTTP header	401 Unauthorized
IT17	Fail to perform a request, because the wrong authentication token is sent in the HTTP header	403 Forbidden

2.2 Simulator

The patient simulator is a Python application that allows to simulate several patients sending simultaneously blood pressure events to the WODIA Web. The aim of it is twofold: 1) simulate several patients so that the WODIA Web's API and UI can be properly verified before deploying the application to actual users; 2) evaluate the performance of the API, so that possible bottlenecks are found before deployment.

To achieve the two aims described above, i.e. test and validate the functionality of the WODIA system, the simulator can be executed in real-time or burst in configuration. The first will set the simulator to operate in real time, i.e. events are sent in the morning and afternoon, as expected when the system is deployed to final users. In burst configuration, the simulator sends, as fast as possible, multiple morning and afternoon events for the number of patients the tester specifies. This mode allows stress test the system and find possible bottlenecks in the Web application and API.

The simulator generates events for both morning and afternoon. Following the blood pressure measurement protocol, these should be performed within a time interval of 10 min, which implies performing a measurement and waiting 1 min between each of the three measurements. This was implemented in the simulator by using a statistical normal distribution to 1) generate a time when the measurements will be performed; and 2) generate blood pressure values, given a blood pressure category (normal, elevated, high blood pressure or hypertensive) attributed to the simulated patient. For point 1, the measurements are generated within a given time window, which, most likely, will be a value in the middle of the interval. For example, for an interval between 6 o'clock and 10 o'clock, in a normal distribution the value will be near 8 o'clock. For point 2, the blood pressure will very likely be a value in the middle of the configured interval. For example, for normal blood pressure, the systolic interval is between 80, 120 mmHg, the generated blood pressure will likely be a value near 100 mmHg.

The events are sent using the WODIA Web HTTP API. It is assumed that this is working as specified, i.e. it complies with the test requirements set in 1. To better simulate a real world scenario, the events are sent in parallel, as if multiple users were performing measurements in the real world.

2.3 Tavern Crawler

This tool is a Visual Studio Code extension that was developed to accelerate the writing of Tavern tests. In short, Tavern tests are written using a custom YAML schema, where each test has a perform and request sections to, respectively, perform a HTTP request to the web server and verify if the response is the expected. Tavern is developed as a pytest plugin, a testing framework for Python. This allows us to use its entire ecosystem. Yet, native support for major Python IDEs such as Visual Studio Code (VSCode) or PyCharm is nonexistent to date, because these only support tests written in Python, which is not the case for Tavern tests which are written in YAML.

For a small number of tests, using the default pytest command line tools for assessing the tests state is easy and fast. The same cannot be stated when the number of tests scale

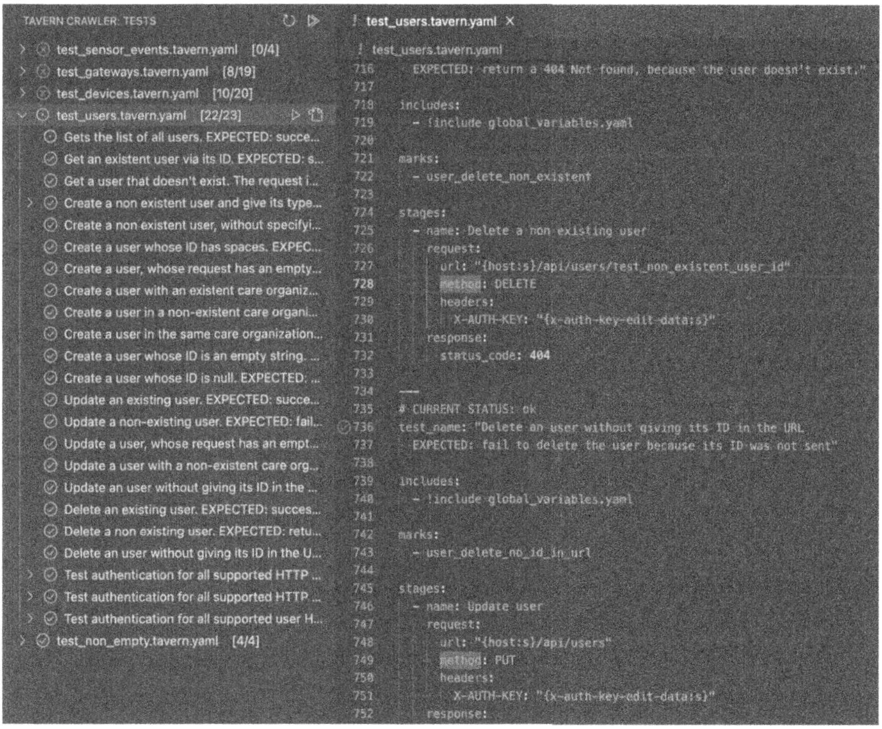

Fig. 4. Panels for the Visual Studio Code's extension Tavern Crawler, which was developed to quickly manage Tavern tests.

to hundreds, which is the case in the WODIA's Web API. The main issues are 1) long text files which can easily reach thousands of lines, making navigation difficult; and 2) the long log formats that makes assessing the issues during writing of the tests and then assessing the results extremely difficult and time consuming. The developed extension, Tavern Crawler, depicted in Fig. 3, initial goals are to ease the navigation through the test files and quickly interpret the test results. This is accomplished by displaying the tests in a tree like navigation menu, along with its known result. In the long term, the aim of the tool is to quickly generate Tavern test files, based in the API description, which can be accomplished if standards such as OpenAPI [16] are used to describe the API (Fig. 4).

3 Results

The total number of integration tests after implementing these with Tavern amounted to 112. A total of 106 tests successfully passed (a total of 6 were failing), corresponding to a 95% pass rate. The issues that made these tests fail are: 1) an issue in the gateways API, where the reference to another entity is made invalid (these totals 1 test); and 2) the device events API are still under development, so the tests are still failing (these total 5 tests).

A burst test with the simulator was also set. This test consisted of 10 simulated patients. For ten days, two blood pressure events, morning, and afternoon, were performed. This amounts to 200 events. The simulation successfully generated and stored the events in the WODIA Web application. This test was repeated ten times and for each of them, all events successfully stored. This was verified visually through the UI and automatically using the HTTP API, specifically by retrieving the events using its ID. In total 2000 events were successfully stored, which is a rate of 100%.

4 Discussion

The results of the integrations tests are successful, although they are still not 100%. Two aspects are worth discussing: 1) the goal of having 100% of passing tests; and 2) how these impacted the interaction between the partners.

For the first aspect, as stated, there is the expectation of having 100% of passing tests, which, at the time of writing, is not the case. The main reason is how the development priorities have been set. As stated, the API must support CRUD requests for devices, device events, gateways, and users. The initial focus was implementing the APIs for devices, gateways, and users, on which device events depend on. Only after these were successfully implemented, the implementation of the device events API started. Because it is still in development, the tests are still failing. Yet, the partners noticed that with this strategy, the assessment of the system was very gradual with little to no rollback necessary. So, it is expected that the development of the device events API benefits from the experience gained and that the goal of 100% is quickly reached.

For the second aspect, having the tests well defined and developing the simulator and the Tavern Crawler extension, aided the writing and assessment of the tests, plus the reporting of errors found between the partners responsible for the development and the test. Having the simulator allowed the different partners to develop the system's components in parallel, especially the gateways that are also still in development. It also allowed to have a preview of how the system might behave once patients start taking and reporting measurements. This is especially important, because problems such as having "dummy" data to thoroughly test the system and technical aspects such as the server's load, could be delayed until the system's actual deployment. The potential consequences of it could be patients' frustration while using the system and eventually leading them to abandon the evaluation, which could lead to poorer experimental results.

The Tavern Crawler extension provided benefits to the test efforts, mostly in assessing and reporting the test results. Right now, the team can be faster reporting issues found in the system, as well as monitoring the development and potential introduction of errors during development. The main potential of a tool like this is in the testing automation. For example, an HTTP API can be specified in a format such as OpenAPI [16]. Having this specification available, an initial set of tests can be automatically generated. This brings advantages to the time that is spent writing the tests and potential errors or lapses that a tester might fail to see.

It is expected that once the gateway is ready, its integration will be fast, because the WODIA Web API, i.e. the interface that connects these components, has already been tested. It is worth referring, as a technical note, that Tavern allows the integration of Python code into the tests. Therefore, the code for the data models that will be used in gateway application, is the same that is being used in the Tavern integration test. This, as a collateral benefit, also validates the implementation of the data models, which can be reported to the gateway development team.

Currently, the limitations of the test methodology and tools are:

- the simulator does not support variation in the category of the blood pressure measurement, i.e. if a simulation runs for 8 weeks, as is expected to happen in the clinical trials, the blood pressure will be the same for this period. Since it is known that 2% of women will present high blood pressure, which might indicate preeclampsia, the simulator could generate a number of patients with this blood pressure variation. The authors expect to implement this feature in the future;
- log-term evaluation of the system using the simulator has not been performed yet, because the WODIA Web component is still under development. Right now, manual tests are enough for reporting major issues, but once these are solved, long term evaluation will start;
- the tools only allow for assessing the WODIA Web API and, currently, there is no integration between the tests performed in the various components, which gives an overview of the overall implementation of the system. For example, it is necessary to replace the simulator with the gateway and test its reliability when sending messages. Knowing the number of messages sent and received, it is possible to investigate any issues that might occur due to, for example, network problems, or issues that were not uncovered during the tests reported in this publication.

5 Conclusion

The WODIA Web API was tested to verify its compliance with the CRUD requests, as well as its reliability and performance. For that existing tools were used and when it was necessary, dedicated tools were developed. Although, currently, the API is not ready, the methodology and techniques used allowed us to measure the progress of the API implementation, which is currently at 95%, and formalize how the measurement is performed during the development of the system. This meets the requirement set acceptance test AT1. Using a simulator allowed to validate the system's reliability and performance (currently 100% of the events are being stored), which meets the requirement set in acceptance test AT2.

Although far from having an integrated and heterogeneous testing platform, these initial blocks enable this goal, as it is possible to test the main integration point. The researchers expect to do this as future work, either by adding more features in Tavern Crawler, by integrating test reporting tools into the development process or by developing more tools that allow test data analysis.

Acknowledgements. This work has been supported by Innovation Fund Denmark (IFD), Denmark, National Centre for Research and Development (NCBR), Poland, Executive Agency for Higher Education, Research, Development and Innovation Funding, (UEFISCDI), Romania in the framework of the ERA PerMed as part of the project WODIA: Personalized Medicine Screening and Monitoring Programme for Pregnant Women Suffering from Preeclampsia and Gestational Hypertension. Also, we would like to say thank you to our clinical collaborators in the WODIA project. Please find more information on WODIA here: https://ece.au.dk/wodia.

References

1. Duley, L.: The global impact of pre-eclampsia and eclampsia. In: Semin Perinatol. **33**(3), 130–137 (2009)
2. Poon, L.C., Magee, L.A., Verlohren, S., Nicolaides, K.H., Shennan, A., von Dadelszen, P., et al.: A literature review and best practice advice for second and third trimester risk stratification, monitoring, and management of pre-eclampsia. In: Int J Gynecol Obstet. **154**(S1), 3–31 (2021)
3. Poon, L.C., Shennan, A., Hyett, J.A., Kapur, A., Hadar, E., Divakar, H., et al.: The international federation of gynecology and obstetrics (FIGO) initiative on pre-eclampsia: a pragmatic guide for first-trimester screening and prevention. In: Int J Gynecol Obstet. **14**(S1), 1–33 (2019)
4. Mazur-Milecka, M., et al.: Preeclampsia risk prediction using machine learning methods trained on synthetic data. In: Strumiłło, P., Klepaczko, A., Strzelecki, M., Bociąga, D. (eds) The Latest Developments and Challenges in Biomedical Engineering. PCBEE 2023. Lecture Notes in Networks and Systems, **746**. Springer, Cham (2024)
5. Pedersen, L., et al.: A time study for the analysis of the potential for the automated stepwise screening program for preeclampsia at week 12 of gestation. International Conference on ICT for Health, Accessibility and Wellbeing. Springer Nature Switzerland, Cham (2022)
6. Wagner, S., Esben, H., Jorge, M.: Demonstration of a micro-services based multi-purpose sensor platform for supporting ambient assisted living systems. In: 12th EAI International Conference on Pervasive Computing Technologies for Healthcare–Demos, Posters, Doctoral Colloquium (2018)

7. Wagner, S.: CARIOT+ care coach–an ambient assisted living ecosystem for supporting open data and open science projects. International Conference on ICT for Health, Accessibility and Wellbeing. Springer International Publishing, Cham (2021)
8. Blood Pressure Service 1.1.1. https://www.bluetooth.com/specifications/specs/blood-pressure-service-1-1-1/. Access 11 Aug 2023
9. Haghi Kashani, M., Madanipour, M., Nikravan, M., Asghari, P., Mahdipour, E.: A systematic review of IoT in healthcare: Applications, techniques, and trends. In: Journal of Network and Computer Applications, **192**, 103164 (2021)
10. Habibzadeh, H., Dinesh, K., Rajabi Shishvan, O., Boggio-Dandry, A., Sharma, G., Soyata, T.: A survey of healthcare internet of things (HIoT): a clinical perspective. In: IEEE Internet of Things J. **7**(1), 53–71 (2020)
11. Hayyolalam, V., Aloqaily, M., Ozkasap, O., Guizani, M.: Edge-assisted solutions for iot-based connected healthcare systems: a literature review. In: IEEE Internet of Things J. **9**(12), 9419–9443 (2022)
12. Bharadwaj, H.K., et al.: A review on the role of machine learning in enabling IoT based healthcare applications. In: IEEE Access **9**, 38859–38890 (2021)
13. Dias, J.P., Couto, F., Paiva, A.C.R., Ferreira, H.S.: A brief overview of existing tools for testing the internet-of-things. In: 2018 IEEE International Conference on Software Testing, Verification and Validation Workshops (ICSTW), pp. 104–109 (2018)
14. Gomez, A.K., Bajaj, S.: Challenges of testing complex internet of things (IoT) devices and systems. In: 2019 11th International Conference on Knowledge and Systems Engineering (KSE), pp. 1–4 (2019)
15. Zhu, S., Yang, S., Gou, X., Xu, Y., Zhang, T., Wan, Y.: Survey of testing methods and testbed development concerning internet of things. In: Wireless Personal Communications **123**(1), 165–194 (2022)
16. OpenAPI. https://www.openapis.org. Access 11 Aug 2023

Transforming Diabetes Care: A Review of IoT-Based Mobile Health Systems

Fiza Ashfaq[1], Abdul Ahad[2,3](✉), Mudassar Hussain[5], and Filipe Madeira[4](✉)

[1] Department of Computer Science, University of Management and Technology, Sialkot 51040, Pakistan

[2] School of Software, Northwestern Polytechnical University, Xian, Shaanxi, People's Republic of China
ahad9388@nwpu.edu.cn

[3] Department of Electronics and Communication Engineering, Istanbul Technical University (ITU), 34467 Istanbul , Turkey

[4] Department of Informatics and Quantitative Methods, Research Center for Arts and Communication (CIAC)/Pole of Digital Literacy and Social Inclusion, Polytechnic Institute of Santarem, 2001-904 Santarem, Portugal
filipe.Madeira@esg.ipsantarem.pt

[5] Department of Computer Science and Creative Technologies, Global College of Engineering and Technology, Muscat, Oman
mudassar.h@gcet.edu.om

Abstract. Diabetes, a chronic ailment requiring ongoing care and monitoring, has undergone a healthcare shift thanks to the Internet of Things (IoT). Real-time monitoring, individualized treatment plans, and improved patient-provider communication are all features of IoT-based mobile health solutions. This study explores the components, functionalities, benefits, and disadvantages of IoT-based mobile health systems for the management of diabetes. It investigates wearable sensors, smartphone apps, and linked devices like glucose meter and monitors, placing a focus on their precision, dependability, and usability. The study explores data analytics techniques that allow for customized advice and actions. Patients can effectively control their diabetes with the use of individualized treatments and real-time monitoring. The research also looks into the data analytical methods used in IoT-based mobile health systems for the treatment of diabetes. IoT-based mobile health system issues and implications are also covered. These include issues with data security and privacy, platform and device compatibility, standardization of data formats, and ensuring that all people with diabetes have equal access to technology. Healthcare workers, academics, and policymakers may learn more about the potential of IoT-based mobile health systems to revolutionize diabetes treatment through this thorough assessment.

Keywords: IoT · Mobile health · Diabetes care · Real-time monitoring · Personalized interventions · Data analytic

---

F. Ashfaq and M. Hussain—Contributing authors.

1 Introduction

Technology and healthcare advancements in recent years have paved the way for revolutionary concepts that might fundamentally alter the way chronic disease treatment is carried out [1]. Healthcare needs and carer needs are expanding disproportionately, with the latter trailing. In addition to the fact that there are more people in the globe, Anderson et al. [2] found that those who use healthcare are living longer. The number of people using mobile phone technology has significantly expanded every year as it has become indispensable. Researchers and medical professionals are utilising the capabilities of mobile phone technology for the benefit of the medical industry [3]. Internet of Things (IoT)-powered mobile health (mHealth) solutions have played a critical role in advancing the area of diabetes treatment to surprising new heights [4]. These Internet of Things (IoT)-based mobile health solutions present a potential strategy to tackle the complicated issues related to managing diabetes, giving people with the disease more control over their condition and raising their general quality of life [5]. Millions of individuals throughout the world suffer from diabetes, a long-term metabolic illness characterised by elevated blood glucose levels. It necessitates ongoing observation, medication management, lifestyle adjustments, and constant interaction with medical professionals [6]. Diabetes management has historically depended significantly on recurrent visits to healthcare institutions, which frequently leads to insufficient surveillance and postponed actions [7]. However, the delivery of diabetes treatment is changing dramatically as a result of the emergence of IoT, the spread of smartphones, and wearable technology [8].

The objective of this study is to investigate the developments and possible advantages of IoT-based mobile health systems for the treatment of diabetes. These systems make real-time monitoring, individualised therapies, and frictionless communication between patients and healthcare professionals possible by utilizing networked devices, sensors, and data analytics. We will evaluate the major elements, features, and results of such systems through a thorough review of previous research studies, shining light on their influence on diabetes self-management and clinical outcomes [9]. There are various benefits of using IoT technology in the treatment of diabetes. It first and foremost makes it possible to remotely and continuously monitor important factors such as blood glucose levels, physical activity, medication adherence, and eating habits. This constant flow of information enables people with diabetes to better understand their status, make wise decisions, and act quickly to avert problems. Additionally, real-time data is available to healthcare professionals, enabling them to provide individualised advice, modify treatment plans, and take aggressive action as required [10].

IoT-based mobile health solutions also promote improved patient participation and self-care. These technologies enable people with diabetes to maintain motivation, follow their treatment programs, and make healthier lifestyle decisions by offering real-time feedback, individualized alerts, and reminders [11]. These systems also encourage patient education by providing instructional materials, interactive technologies, and social support networks, which develop a feeling of community and information exchange among people with diabetes. This research focuses on the use of IoT-based mobile health systems for the management of diabetes. The goal is to give a thorough review of the characteristics, advantages, difficulties, and directions these systems are headed in the future [12].

This research also examines the difficulties and restrictions related to the use of IoT-based mobile health systems in treating diabetes. We seek to give a thorough knowledge of the constraints that need to be overcome for general use and acceptance of these systems by critically exploring topics including data security, privacy concerns, interoperability, and equity of access. Figure 1: Shows the Architecture for Diabetes Patients Monitoring. Finally, this study suggests prospective research treatments and future prospects for IoT-based mobile health systems for the treatment of diabetes. We hope to contribute to these systems' continuous development and improvement by highlighting gaps in the existing literature and outlining potential topics for additional research [13].

1.1 Research Questions

1. How do IoT-based mobile health systems affect the standard of treatment and outcomes for diabetics in terms of health?
2. What difficulties and obstacles are related to the acceptance and application of IoT-based mobile health systems in the treatment of diabetes?
3. What categories of Internet of Things (IoT) products and technologies are most frequently used in the treatment of diabetes, and how successful are they in actual use cases?
4. How do people with diabetes and healthcare professionals interact with and view IoT-based mobile health solutions for managing their condition?
5. What ethical and privacy issues are involved in gathering and exploiting patient data for IoT-based diabetic care?

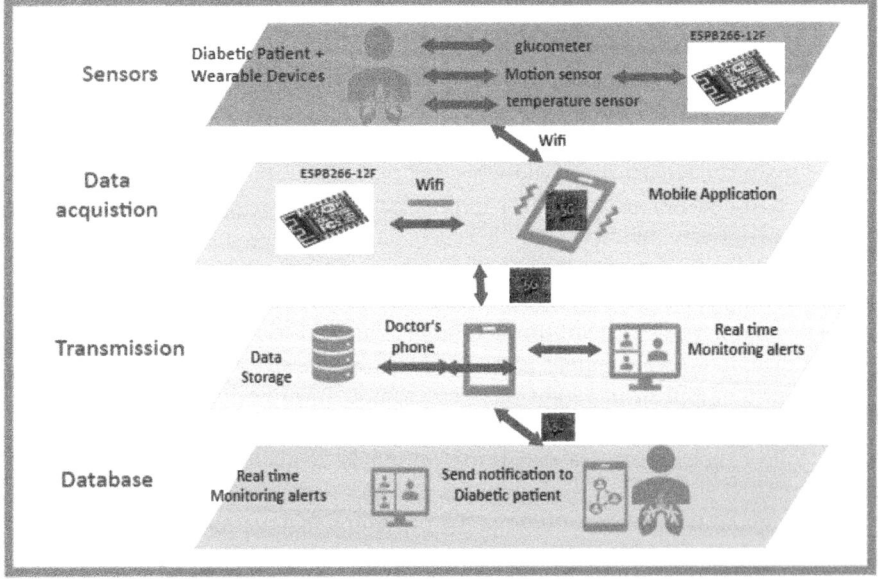

Fig. 1. Architecture for Diabetes Patients Monitoring

1.2 Our Contribution

With a thorough examination of the role that IoT-based mobile health systems have played in modernising diabetes treatment, this review article intends to add to the body of knowledge already available. While earlier research has examined the advantages and drawbacks of these systems, this study offers a distinctive viewpoint by highlighting the part played by patients as active participants in their own treatment and the possibilities for customized therapies. The analysis of how well IoT-based mobile health systems perform in terms of enhancing patient outcomes is one of the paper's main contributions. We seek to give evidence-based insights into the influence of these systems on important diabetes management variables such as glycemic control, medication adherence, and lifestyle adjustments by synthesizing and analyzing the findings of prior research studies.

1.3 Organization of this Paper

The remaining paper is arranged, as follows. In Sect. 2, the Literature review is defined. Internet of Things-based mobile health systems for diabetes are covered in Sect. 3, and Aware m-health systems are covered in Sect. 4. Recent studies on Transforming Diabetes Care are discussed in Sect. 5. The challenges and elements of Internet-based m-health systems for diabetes are discussed in Sect. 6. Comparing various diabetes management methods is covered in Sect. 7. The paper's conclusion is provided in the next and last part, which also includes some new suggestions for further research.

2 Literature Review

The paper [14], "An IoT-based Foot Healthcare System for Diabetic Patients and a Futuristic Approach for Transforming Sensor Data into Real-time Medical Advice" is a critical evaluation and study of the relevant literature, research, and studies that are already available on the subject. In this instance, the review's objective is to examine the level of knowledge and technological developments in relation to IoT-based foot healthcare systems for diabetic patients, with an emphasis on how sensor data may be used to deliver real-time medical guidance.

The research article [15], "An advanced conceptual diagnostic healthcare framework for diabetes and cardiovascular disorders" is a thorough and methodical investigation of the creation and use of improved diagnostic healthcare systems for cardiovascular and diabetic problems. This kind of literature review tries to provide readers with a complete picture of the status of the field's knowledge and recent developments.

A study article [16], "IoT-based healthcare systems: A survey" gives a thorough review of the current state of IoT-based healthcare systems, highlighting their uses, advantages, difficulties, and opportunities for the future.

The research paper [17], "Analysis of factors affecting IoT-based smart hospital design" gives a thorough awareness of the numerous factors to take into account and the difficulties to be faced while developing IoT-based smart healthcare settings. Offers significant insights for healthcare professionals, academics, and policymakers involved in smart healthcare projects by providing a thorough review of the elements that influence the design and implementation of IoT-based smart hospitals.

The paper [18], "Recent trends and advances in type 1 diabetes therapeutics: A comprehensive review" concerning the most current developments and developing trends in the management of Type 1 diabetes. aims to give readers a thorough overview of the most recent advancements in Type 1 diabetes therapy, including cutting-edge medications, equipment, and scientific discoveries.

A study article [19], "Glucose-activatable insulin delivery with charge-conversional polyelectrolyte multilayers for diabetes care" involving the creation and use of charge-conversional polyelectrolyte multilayers in glucose-activatable insulin delivery systems. To offer a thorough grasp of the technological and scientific features, possible applications, and ramifications of this novel method of treating diabetes.

The research article [20], "Emerging Diabetes Technologies: Continuous Glucose Monitors/Artificial Pancreases" is an in-depth analysis of the most recent innovations and breakthroughs in diabetes treatment, concentrating on continuous glucose monitors (CGMs) and artificial pancreases. This offers a thorough overview of the technical, scientific, and medical elements of these cutting-edge diabetic treatments. Gives a thorough review of the most recent advancements and clinical uses of artificial pancreas and continuous glucose monitors in the treatment of diabetes. It is a helpful tool for researchers, medical professionals, and people with diabetes who want to comprehend and efficiently use this new technology.

Tables 1, 2, and 3 provides a detail overview on the existing papers related to the topic.

Table 1. Summary of the existing schemes.

Ref	Year	Title	Objectives	Advantages
[14]	2022	An IoT-based Foot Healthcare System for Diabetic Patients and a Futuristic Approach for transforming Sensor Data into real-time Medical Advice	The study's futuristic methodology relies on technology to deliver prompt and individualised medical advice, thereby raising the standard of care for diabetic patients as a whole.	Patients have a priceless tool for managing diabetes, which ultimately improves patient outcomes, lowers healthcare costs, and raises the standard of treatment as a whole.
[15]	2019	An advanced conceptual diagnostic healthcare framework for diabetes and cardiovascular disorders	To enhance the early diagnosis and treatment of cardiovascular and diabetic diseases. The creation and validation of the framework are essential steps towards raising the standard of treatment, lowering healthcare expenditures, and promoting the general health of people with certain chronic diseases.	The management of diabetes and cardiovascular illnesses may be improved with the use of an advanced conceptual diagnostic healthcare framework, which will eventually benefit patients, healthcare professionals, and the larger healthcare ecosystem.

3 Internet of Things-Based Mobile Health Systems for Diabetes

IoT-based mobile health (m-health) systems have become a potential strategy for managing diabetes, giving a number of advantages and chances for better care. Real-time monitoring, individualized therapies, and improved patient interaction are made possible by these systems by utilizing networked devices, sensors, and data analytics. The components and benefits of IoT-based m-health solutions for diabetes are covered in this article [21]. One of the key features of IoT-based mobile health systems for diabetes is their capability to collect and interpret real-time data. Connected gadgets like glucose metres, insulin pumps, and wearable sensors provide continuous monitoring of blood glucose levels, activity levels, sleep patterns, and other crucial factors. The collection of real-time data offers informative data on a patient's health, allowing for personalized treatments and therapy adjustments [22].

3.1 Monitoring in Real-Time

IoT-enabled gadgets, including wearable sensors and continuous glucose monitors (CGMs), offer real-time information on blood sugar levels, activity levels, sleep cycles, and other crucial factors. Through continuous monitoring, diabetic patients and their medical professionals can identify patterns in the data and make prompt treatment changes [23].

3.2 Customised Interventions

Mobile apps and linked devices are used by IoT-based m-health systems to deliver personalised therapies. Medication adherence reminders, alerts for blood glucose levels, suggestions for physical activity, and food monitoring are some of these treatments [24]. These technologies enable patients to take control of their illness and make well-informed decisions by customizing therapies to their specific requirements.

3.3 Improvements in Patient Engagement

IoT-based m-health solutions encourage patient participation with the use of engaging mobile apps and networked gadgets. Patients have access to peer support networks, self-management tools, and educational materials. Patients who can actively engage in their treatment are more empowered and have a better grasp of managing their diabetes, which results in improved adherence and outcomes [23].

3.4 Remote Observation and Telemedicine

IoT-based m-health systems offer remote monitoring of patient health data, enabling healthcare practitioners to analyse and react to changes in real time.

This remote monitoring lessens the requirement for frequent in-person clinic visits, increases access to treatment, and improves patient convenience. Virtual consultations are another feature of telemedicine that promotes the ongoing connection between patients and medical professionals [25].

Table 2. Summary of the existing reviews

Ref	Year	Title	Objectives	Advantages
[16]	2019	IoT-based healthcare systems: A survey	In order to fully understand IoT-based healthcare systems, their influence on healthcare delivery, and the potential and problems they provide in the dynamic healthcare environment.	To show how IoT-based healthcare solutions have the power to revolutionise patient care, healthcare delivery, and the healthcare sector as a whole.
[17]	2022	Analysis of factors affecting IoT-based smart hospital design	Ensure that IoT-based smart hospitals efficiently utilise IoT technology to improve patient care, streamline operations, and boost overall healthcare outcomes while taking into account the related problems and concerns.	the significance of doing an extensive examination of aspects influencing IoT-based smart hospital design, as it can lead to more effective, patient-centred, and technologically advanced healthcare facilities.
[18]	2023	Recent trends and advances in type 1 diabetes therapeutics: A comprehensive review	emphasise the need of being informed on the most recent advancements in type 1 diabetes therapies and sharing this knowledge to improve patient care and results.	By enhancing understanding, treatment choices, and overall diabetes care, healthcare professionals and patients can both benefit.
[19]	2022	Glucose-activatable insulin delivery with charge-conversational polyelectrolyte multilayers for diabetes care	the potential for charge-conversational polyelectrolyte multilayers in glucose-activatable insulin delivery systems to revolutionise the treatment of diabetes and enhance the quality of life for those with the condition.	Delivery of glucose-activatable insulin via charge-conversational polyelectrolyte multilayers is expected to revolutionise the treatment of diabetes, boost patient outcomes, and generally improve the quality of life for those with the condition.

Table 3. Summary of the existing schemes.

Ref	Year	Title	Objectives	Advantages
[20]	2023	Emerging Diabetes Technologies: Continuous Glucose Monitors/Artificial Pancreases	to enhance the lives of people with diabetes and advance the area of diabetes treatment by using the potential of Continuous Glucose Monitors and Artificial Pancreases.	emphasise the potential of CGMs and Artificial pancreas to revolutionise diabetes treatment, boost patient outcomes, and ultimately improve the lives of persons with diabetes.
[20]	2023	Emerging Diabetes Technologies: Continuous Glucose Monitors/Artificial Pancreases	to enhance the lives of people with diabetes and advance the area of diabetes treatment by using the potential of Continuous Glucose Monitors and Artificial Pancreases.	emphasise the potential of CGMs and Artificial pancreas to revolutionise diabetes treatment, boost patient outcomes, and ultimately improve the lives of persons with diabetes.

3.5 Remote Observation and Telemedicine

The IoT infrastructure makes it easier to gather, store, and analyze vast amounts of health data. These data sets may be subjected to advanced analytics treatments in order to find trends, correlations, and insights that support individualized diabetes care [5]. The use of data-driven decision-making facilitates the creation of prediction models for the early identification and avoidance of issues.

3.6 More Effective Healthcare Coordination

Healthcare providers may communicate and share patient data more easily thanks to IoT-based m-health technologies. Comprehensive patient profiles and a holistic approach to therapy are made possible by the integration of data from several sources, including wearable technology, electronic health records, and CGMs [26]. By enhancing coordination, information gaps are less likely to occur and group decision-making is encouraged.

3.7 Adaptability and the Ability to Scale

Due to the extensive use of mobile devices and internet access, m-health solutions based on the IoT offer the potential for broad acceptance and scalability. These systems can reach a broader population, including under-served regions, bridging diabetes treatment gaps and improving equity in access to healthcare services [27], IoT-based m-health solutions can transform diabetes care. These technologies have the potential to revolutionise diabetes management through real-time monitoring, customised therapies, greater patient participation, remote monitoring, data analytics, and better healthcare coordination. By using IoT technology, we can develop cutting-edge solutions that improve patient outcomes, provide people with diabetes with more control over their condition, and raise the standard of care as a whole.

4 Aware M-Health Systems

A mobile health system that is "aware" is one that has awareness capabilities [28]. It implies that the system can collect information about its users and their surroundings, analyze that information, and utilize it to deliver personalized and context-aware services and interventions [29]. This concept combines a number of technologies, including sensors, data analytics, and artificial intelligence, to build a more intelligent and responsive m-health system. An m-health system's awareness capabilities may include the following:

4.1 Contextual Knowledge

To give personalized treatments, the system may gather and analyse contextual data such as location, time, activity level, and environmental elements. It can, for example, send medicine or exercise reminders based on the user's present environment [30].

4.2 Personalized Interventions

An alert m-health system may deliver personalized suggestions, reminders, and alerts by using user data and preferences. It considers individual traits, health objectives, and historical data to give therapies tailored to each user's requirements.

4.3 Adaptive Learning

An intelligent m-health system may continually learn from user interactions and feedback to enhance its services over time [27]. It may tailor its suggestions and interventions depending on the user's reactions and preferences, resulting in a more personalized and successful experience.

4.4 Proactive Monitoring

An aware m-health system, rather than depending exclusively on user-initiated actions, may actively monitor user data and flag potential health concerns or deviations from usual trends. It can then send proactive warnings or alerts to the user or their healthcare practitioner [31].

4.5 Intelligent Suggestions

Using powerful analytics and machine learning algorithms, an intelligent m-health system may provide intelligent insights and actionable suggestions based on the user's data [32]. It can find patterns, trends, and correlations in data, allowing for improved health outcomes and more informed decision-making. The concept of an aware m-health system has great potential for increasing the efficacy and user experience of mobile health services [25]. By leveraging the power of awareness and intelligent technology, these systems may provide more personalised, responsive, and proactive healthcare services, ultimately leading to improved patient outcomes and a higher level of engagement in self-care.

5 Recent Studies on Transforming Diabetes Care: A Review of IoT-Based Mobile Health Systems

I'll give a broad overview of the areas that researchers often concentrate on when researching the use of IoT in healthcare for monitoring diabetes patients, as well as some frequent issues with these studies. The main goals of research in this area are to examine and assess the viability, efficacy, and possible advantages of employing IoT technology for controlling and monitoring diabetes [33]. Their work frequently entails Research Review: To assess the present status of IoT technologies in diabetes care, identify knowledge gaps, and create the study environment, researchers evaluate the body of existing literature.

- **Design and Implementation of Systems:** IoT-based platforms or systems are created and developed by researchers with a focus on managing and monitoring diabetes. In order to gather and send pertinent health data, this may include the integration of multiple devices, sensors, and communication technologies [30].
- **Information Gathering and Analysis:** Researchers use IoT devices and sensors to gather real-time or historical data from diabetes patients. They examine the data collected to learn more about the condition of the patients, the effectiveness of the treatments, and the course of the diseases [34].
- **Analysis of Performance:** Researchers consider the quality and dependability of the data, the timeliness of the data transfer, the user experience, and the system efficiency when evaluating the performance of an IoT-based system. To determine benefits or drawbacks, they might assess how the IoT-based system performs in comparison to more conventional healthcare methods [27].
- **Clinical Results and Patient Experience:** Researchers investigate how IoT-based monitoring affects healthcare results and patient satisfaction. This entails assessing enhancements in blood glucose management, problems being reduced, patient happiness, quality of life, and self-management skills.

– **Analyses of Cost-Effectiveness:** In order to treat diabetes, researchers examine the economic viability and cost-effectiveness of adopting IoT-based monitoring systems. This entails taking into account elements including the initial setup expenses, ongoing maintenance costs, and prospective healthcare cost savings and treatment of problems associated with diabetes [35].

Table 4. Summary of treatments, objectives, performance measures, requirements and communication technologies of Transforming Diabetes Care: A Review of IoT-Based Mobile Health Systems that proposed in this paper

Treatments	Objectives	Performance Measures	Communication Technologies
Continuous Glucose Monitoring (CGM) Systems	Improve Glucose Monitoring and Control	Glycemic Control	Sensor Devices
Wearable Devices	Enhance Medication Adherence	Medication Adherence	Connectivity
Mobile Applications	Facilitate Lifestyle Modifications	User Engagement	Data Security and Privacy
Telemedicine and Remote Monitoring	Enable Remote Patient Monitoring	Patient Satisfaction	Interoperability
Data Analytics and Machine Learning	Empower Patients	Health Outcomes	User-Friendly Interfaces

6 The Challenges and Elements of Internet-Based M-Health Systems for Diabetes

Diabetes m-health systems that are internet-based confront a number of difficulties and need to carefully take into account a number of factors in order to be implemented. The following are some significant difficulties and factors to take into account:

6.1 Data Privacy and Security

It is critical to safeguard the confidentiality and privacy of patient data. Internet-based mobile health systems must employ strong security measures to prevent unauthorized access to or breaches of critical health information. Data security is mostly dependent on encryption, safe data storage, user authentication, and adherence to privacy laws [36]. Numerous prospects for real-time monitoring, improved communication, and customised interventions are opened up by the use of IoT-based mobile health systems in the management of diabetes. However, it also puts a wealth of confidential patient data in danger. Strong security measures must be put in place to guarantee the confidentiality and integrity of patient data.

The defences that prevent unauthorised access include encryption techniques, safe data storage, and strict user authentication procedures. It is not just a legal necessity, but also a moral obligation to uphold patient rights, and to comply with healthcare privacy laws like HIPAA and GDPR [37]. The safety of the Internet and patient privacy are the two main issues that need to be addressed while using them. Different parts of the globe uphold privacy rules to safeguard the privacy of patients [37]. The General Data Protection Regulation (GDPR) in Europe and the Health Insurance Portability and Accountability Act (HIPAA) in the United States, for instance, set these. In order to give more security, the most current authenticated key agreement systems for HIPAA and GDPR privacy/security use modular exponential computations or scalar multiplications on elliptic curves, however they are computationally intensive and hence expensive to implement [38]. Figure 2: illustrates the impact of IoT on health.

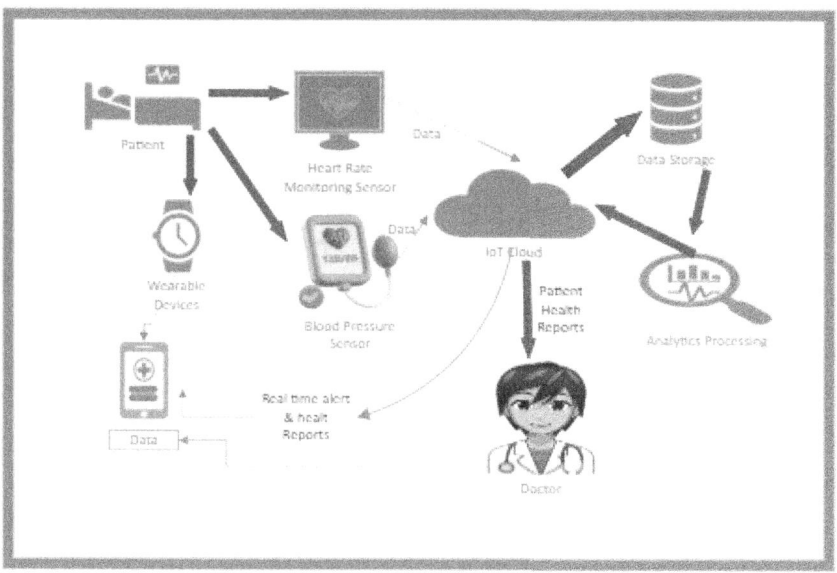

Fig. 2. Impact of IoT on health.

6.2 Interoperability

The seamless interchange of data and integration of many platforms, devices, and healthcare systems depend on interoperability. To enable interoperability and efficient data sharing between different elements of the m-health system, such as glucose monitors, mobile applications, electronic health records, and healthcare provider systems, standardization of data formats, communication protocols, and interoperability frameworks is essential [39]. Table 4: shows the Summary of treatments, objectives, performance measures, requirements and communication technologies of Transforming Diabetes Care: A Review of IoT-Based Mobile Health Systems proposed in this paper.

6.3 Infrastructure and Accessibility

Systematic internet access is crucial for internet-based mobile health applications. However, the limited availability of dependable internet connectivity, particularly in rural or distant places, may prevent the broad adoption of these systems. For effective communication and data transfer, it is essential to have a sufficient network infrastructure, including broadband internet and mobile networks.

6.4 Barriers to Access and the Digital Divide

The term "digital divide" describes differences in how accessible technology and online services are to certain communities. Affordability of devices, digital literacy, language obstacles, and usability for people with different backgrounds and abilities should all be taken into account when designing internet-based m-health solutions. Addressing these gaps and providing fair access to m-health solutions are necessary to close the digital divide [40].

6.5 Acceptance and Involvement of Users

User acceptability and involvement are essential for the achievement of internet-based mobile health systems. User adoption and long-term engagement may be increased by creating intuitive mobile applications, user-friendly user interfaces, and compelling features. To encourage user adoption as well as adherence to the system, it is essential to take into account user preferences, requirements, and comments during the designing and deployment processes [41].

6.6 Workflow and Integration of Health Systems

Internet-based m-health solutions must be integrated into current healthcare processes for effective care coordination and teamwork. The workflows of healthcare providers, clinical decision support tools, and electronic health record systems should all be compatible with these systems. For integration into the healthcare system to be effective, it is also essential to be in compliance with healthcare laws, rules, and reimbursement models.

6.7 Dependability and Technical Assistance

Systems for mobile health that are dependent on the Internet must be dependable, robust, and backed by effective technical support. To guarantee system stability and performance, regular upkeep, upgrades, and monitoring are required.

For resolving any technical difficulties and guaranteeing customer happiness, it's critical to offer enough technical support, troubleshooting techniques, and user help channels.

6.8 Review and Evidence-Based Practise

Internet-based m-health solutions should be thoroughly researched and reviewed in order to determine their effectiveness, safety, and usability. Evidence-based insights into how these systems affect diabetes care and patient outcomes may be obtained by conducting clinical trials, user studies, and outcome assessments. For refining and optimising system functioning, user feedback must be taken into account, and research findings must be continuously improved [33]. Internet-based m-health systems for diabetes can overcome obstacles and offer efficient, available, and secure solutions for diabetes management and treatment by addressing these issues and taking into account these factors.

7 Comparing Various Diabetes Management Methods

Monitoring of blood glucose levels, keeping track of medication and lifestyle choices, and making well-informed decisions are all important tasks for people with diabetes. Diabetes management systems play a critical part in this process. Numerous diabetes management systems are available, each with unique features and capabilities. Following is a comparison of several diabetes control methods.

7.1 Logbooks Traditionally Created on Paper

Features: A straightforward and low-tech approach for keeping track of insulin dosages, food consumption, and blood glucose levels. Benefits include affordability, usability, and accessibility. Cons: Requires manual computations and has limited trend tracking and data analysis capabilities [42].

7.2 Blood Glucose Monitor with Manual Tracking

Features: A glucose meter has the capacity to manually log pertinent information, including blood glucose measurements. Advantages: Accurate blood glucose readings are provided, and manual tracking of medication, diet, and exercise is possible. Cons: Manual data entry is required, limited data analysis capabilities, and risk of human error.

7.3 Mobile Applications for Diabetes

Features: Programs created particularly for managing diabetes on mobile devices. Pros: include simple data entry, automated glucose measurement collection (if a glucose meter is supported), data analysis, and trend tracking. Cons: Dependence on human input, potential accuracy issues if not synchronised with a trustworthy glucose metre and varied degrees of usefulness among applications.

Table 5. Comparing various diabetes management methods

Performance	Web Based System	Robot Assisted system	Smart phone assisted system	Interactive Mhealth-System
Cost	Low	High	medium	medium
Security	insecure	secure	secure	secure
Complexity	Low	High	medium	medium
Protocols Used	GPRS	GPRS, Wi-Fi	GPRS-Bluetooth,	PRS, XML, MQTT
Flexibility	No	Yes	Yes,	Yes
User Interaction with system	No	Yes	Yes,	Yes
User Control over system	No	No	Yes,	Yes

7.4 (CGM) Systems for Continuous Glucose Monitoring

Features: CGM systems deliver data from a sensor that continually measures blood sugar levels to a receiver or smartphone [43]. The interaction with insulin pumps and mobile applications, trend analysis, alarms for high and low glucose levels, and real-time glucose measurements are all positive features. Cons: Higher cost, a chance for errors, the necessity for calibration, and the requirement for replacing and reinstalling sensors. Table 5 shows the Comparison of various diabetes management methods

7.5 Diabetes Integrated Management Systems

Features: Complete platforms or devices that integrate glucose monitoring, insulin administration, and data analysis. Advantages include real-time glucose monitoring, automatic insulin administration, data analysis, trend tracking, and individualised suggestions. Cons: Higher price, difficult setup and upkeep, risk for technological problems, and restricted availability. When contrasting various diabetes management systems, it's crucial to take into account elements like precision, practicality, data analysis skills, platform or device integration, price, user-friendliness, and personal preferences. The best method for each person may also be chosen by speaking with healthcare experts and taking into account their particular requirements and aspirations. It is important to note that the field of diabetes management systems is quickly developing as a result of technological improvements and the introduction of new products. Making decisions on diabetes care, therefore, requires keeping up with the most recent discoveries and finding out new information.

8 Conclusions and Future Work

8.1 Conclusions

In short, this study has given a thorough overview of IoT-based mobile health (m-health) solutions that are revolutionizing the way that diabetes treatment is delivered. The analysis highlights the IoT-based mobile health systems transforming the potential for diabetes care. These technologies provide groundbreaking approaches to real-time monitoring, individualised care, and enhanced patient outcomes. By obtaining access to extensive patient data, IoT technologies help the healthcare industry by facilitating more precise diagnoses, individualised treatment plans, and quick interventions. Delivery of healthcare might become more effective and efficient as a result. IoT-based mobile health solutions are a paradigm change in the way that diabetes is handled, to sum up. They may greatly raise the standard of living for diabetics and increase the effectiveness of healthcare services. We have emphasized the traits, advantages, difficulties, and directions these systems should go in the future.

By incorporating IoT technology into diabetes treatment, healthcare delivery might be revolutionised, with better patient outcomes and higher standards of care all around. Personalized therapies, real-time blood glucose monitoring, and improved patient involvement are all made possible by IoT-based mobile health solutions. These systems enable people with diabetes to take an active role in managing their disease and make well-informed decisions by utilizing networked devices, sensors, and data analytics. The remote monitoring capabilities and telemedicine functionalities of these systems also enhance communication and collaboration between patients and healthcare providers, leading to more efficient and timely interventions. However, several challenges need to be addressed for the successful implementation and widespread adoption of IoT-based m-health systems for diabetes care. Data security and privacy concerns, interoperability among different devices and platforms, connectivity and infrastructure limitations, and the digital divide are important considerations. This study also shows that the suggested system is very computationally efficient and in compliance with GDPR privacy principles and HIPAA privacy/security laws.

8.2 Future-Work

More research and development efforts are required in the future to enhance IoT-based m-health systems for diabetes treatment. Here are some possible future projects:

1. Enhancements to security and privacy
2. Standardisation and Interoperability
3. Accessibility and scalability
4. Usability and User Experience
5. Evidence Generation and Clinical Validation

Integration with Artificial Intelligence and Machine Learning: By focusing on these areas of future research, we can continue to transform diabetes care through IoT-based m-health systems, resulting in improved patient outcomes, improved self-management, and a more patient-centric approach to healthcare delivery.

Acknowledgment:. This work is funded by national funds through FCT - Foundation for Science and Technology, I.P., under project UIDP/04019/2020.

References

1. Ahad, A., Tahir, M.: Perspective-6g and IoT for intelligent healthcare: challenges and future research directions. ECS Sensors Plus **2**(1), 011601 (2023)
2. Anderson, K., Burford, O., Emmerton, L.: Mobile health apps to facilitate self-care: a qualitative study of user experiences. PLoS ONE **11**(5), e0156164 (2016)
3. Ahad, A., et al.: A comprehensive review on 5g-based smart healthcare network security: taxonomy, issues, solutions and future research directions. In: Array, p. 100290 (2023)
4. Stephen, B.U.-A., Uzoewulu, B.C., Asuquo, P.M., Ozuomba, S.: Diabetes and hypertension mobilehealth systems: a review of general challenges and advancements. J. Eng. Appl. Sci. **70**(1), 78 (2023)
5. Deshkar, S., Thanseeh, R., Menon, V.G.: A review on IoT based m-health systems for diabetes. Int. J. Comput. Sci. Telecommun. **8**(1), 13–18 (2017)
6. Ahad, A., Tahir, M., Sheikh, M.A.S., Mughees, A., Ahmed, K.I.: Optimal route selection in 5g-based smart health-care network: a reinforcement learning approach. In: 2021 26th IEEE Asia-Pacific Conference on Communications (APCC), pp. 248–253. IEEE (2021)
7. Al-Rawashdeh, M., Keikhosrokiani, P., Belaton, B., Alawida, M., Zwiri, A.: Iot adoption and application for smart healthcare: a systematic review. Sensors **22**(14), 5377 (2022)
8. Ahad, A., Tahir, M., Sheikh, M.A.S., Hassan, N., Ahmed, K.I., Mughees, A.: A game theory based clustering scheme (GCS) for 5g-based smart healthcare. In: IEEE 5th International Symposium on Telecommunication Technologies (ISTT), pp. 157–161. IEEE (2020)
9. Goyal, S., Sharma, N., Bhushan, B., Shankar, A., Sagayam, M.: Iot enabled technology in secured healthcare: applications, challenges and future directions. In: Cognitive Internet of Medical Things for Smart Healthcare: Services and Applications, pp. 25–48 (2021)
10. de Neira, A.B., Kantarci, B., Nogueira, M.: Distributed denial of service attack prediction: challenges, open issues and opportunities. Comput. Netw. **222**, 109553 (2023)
11. Ahmed, M., Byreddy, S., Nutakki, A., Sikos, L.F., Haskell-Dowland, P.: ECU-IOHT: a dataset for analyzing cyberattacks in internet of health things. Ad Hoc Netw. **122**, 102621 (2021)
12. Chang, S.-H., Chiang, R.-D., Wu, S.-J., Chang, W.-T.: A context-aware, interactive m-health system for diabetics. IT Professional **18**(3), 14–22 (2016)
13. Almotiri, S.H., Khan, M.A., Alghamdi, M.A.: Mobile health (m-health) system in the context of IoT. In: IEEE 4th International Conference on Future Internet of Things and Cloud Workshops (FiCloudW), pp. 39–42. IEEE (2016)

14. Mydhili, S., SK, D.M., Naseera, F., Kumar, R., et al.: An IoT based foot healthcare system for diabetic patients and a futuristic approach for transforming sensor data into real-time medical advice. In: Proceedings of the Advancement in Electronics and Communication Engineering (2022)
15. Sharma, M., Singh, G., Singh, R.: An advanced conceptual diagnostic healthcare framework for diabetes and cardiovascular disorders. arXiv preprint arXiv:1901.10530 (2019)
16. Yassein, M.B., Hmeidi, I., Al-Harbi, M., Mrayan, L., Mardini, W., Khamayseh, Y.: IoT-based healthcare systems: a survey. In: Proceedings of the Second International Conference on Data Science, E-Learning and Information Systems, pp. 1–9 (2019)
17. Uslu, B.Ç., Okay, E., Dursun, E.: Analysis of factors affecting IoT-based smart hospital design. J. Cloud Comput. **9**(1), 1–23 (2020)
18. Singh, A., et al.: Recent trends and advances in type 1 diabetes therapeutics: a comprehensive review. Eur. J. Cell Biol. **102**(2), 151329 (2023)
19. Yang, Y., Wang, X., Yuan, X., Zhu, Q., Chen, S., Xia, D.: Glucose-activatable insulin delivery with charge-conversional polyelectrolyte multilayers for diabetes care. Front. Bioeng. Biotechnol. **10**, 996763 (2022)
20. Almurashi, A.M., Rodriguez, E., Garg, S.K.: Emerging diabetes technologies: continuous glucose monitors/artificial pancreases. J. Indian Inst. Sci. **103**(1), 205–230 (2023)
21. Mishra, K.N., Chakraborty, C.: A novel approach towards using big data and IoT for improving the efficiency of m-health systems. In: Advanced Computational Intelligence Techniques for Virtual Reality in Healthcare, pp. 123–139 (2020)
22. Veena, A., Gowrishankar, S.: Applications, opportunities, and current challenges in the healthcare industry. In: IoT in Healthcare Systems, pp. 121–147. CRC Press (2023)
23. Gómez, J., Oviedo, B., Zhuma, E.: Patient monitoring system based on internet of things. Procedia Comput. Sci. **83**, 90–97 (2016)
24. Lee, K., et al.: Diffusion of a lifelog-based digital healthcare platform for future precision medicine: data provision and verification study. J. Personaliz. Med. **12**(5), 803 (2022)
25. Huang, J., Wu, X., Huang, W., Wu, X., Wang, S.: Internet of things in health management systems: a review. Int. J. Commun. Syst. **34**(4), e4683 (2021)
26. Ahsan, M.J.: Future challenges of IOMT applications. In: Security and Privacy Issues in Internet of Medical Things, pp. 117–132. Elsevier (2023)
27. Farooq, M.S., Riaz, S., Tehseen, R., Farooq, U., Saleem, K.: Role of internet of things in diabetes healthcare: network infrastructure, taxonomy, challenges, and security model. Digital health **9**, 20552076231179056 (2023)
28. Mandari, H., Yahaya, M.: Examining factors influencing intention to use m-health applications for promoting healthier life among smartphone users in tanzania. J. Int. Technol. Inf. Manag. **31**(2), 1–21 (2022)
29. Qadri, Y.A., Nauman, A., Zikria, Y.B., Vasilakos, A.V., Kim, S.W.: The future of healthcare internet of things: a survey of emerging technologies. IEEE Commun. Surv. Tutor. **22**(2), 1121–1167 (2020)
30. Rahman, R.A., Aziz, N.S.A., Kassim, M., Yusof, M.I.: Iot-based personal health care monitoring device for diabetic patients. In: IEEE Symposium on Computer Applications & Industrial Electronics (ISCAIE), vol. 2017, pp. 168–173. IEEE (2017)
31. Subhan, F., et al.: AI-enabled wearable medical internet of things in healthcare system: a survey. Appl. Sci. **13**(3), 1394 (2023)

32. Butt, H.A., et al.: Federated machine learning in 5g smart healthcare: a security perspective review. Procedia Comput. Sci. **224**, 580–586 (2023)
33. Chhabra, P.: Issues and challenges associated with machine learning tools for health care system: a review. NEU J. Artif. Intell. Internet of Things **2**(2) (2023)
34. Albahri, A.S., et al.: IoT-based telemedicine for disease prevention and health promotion: state-of-the-art. J. Netw. Comput. Appl. **173**, 102873 (2021)
35. Menon, S.P., et al.: An intelligent diabetic patient tracking system based on machine learning for e-health applications. Sensors **23**(6), 3004 (2023)
36. Ahad, A., Tahir, M., Sheikh, M.A., Ahmed, K.I., Mughees, A.: An intelligent clustering-based routing protocol (CRP-GR) for 5g-based smart healthcare using game theory and reinforcement learning. Appl. Sci. **11**(21), 9993 (2021)
37. Lee, T.-F., Chang, I.-P., Su, G.-J.: Compliance with hipaa and gdpr in certificateless-based authenticated key agreement using extended chaotic maps. Electronics **12**(5), 1108 (2023)
38. Essefi, I., Rahmouni, H.B., Solomonides, T., Ladeb, M.F.: Hipaa controlled patient information exchange and traceability in clinical processes. In: 2022 IEEE 9th International Conference on Sciences of Electronics, Technologies of Information and Telecommunications (SETIT), pp. 452–460. IEEE (2022)
39. Rayan, R.A., Zafar, I., Tsagkaris, C., Papazoglou, A.S., Moysidis, D.V.: Pervasive m-health for chronic diseases. In: Computational Intelligence for Medical Internet of Things (MIoT) Applications, pp. 301–314 (2023)
40. Devi, D.H., et al.: 5G technology in healthcare and wearable devices: a review. Sensors **23**(5), 2519 (2023)
41. Ahad, A., Al Faisal, S., Ali, F., Jan, B., Ullah, N., et al.: Design and performance analysis of DSS (Dual Sink Based Scheme) protocol for WBASNS. Adv. Remote Sens. **6**(04), 245 (2017)
42. Raikar, A.S., Kumar, P., Raikar, G.V.S., Somnache, S.N.: Advances and challenges in IoT-based smart drug delivery systems: a comprehensive review. Appl. Syst. Innov. **6**(4), 62 (2023)
43. Ayesha, A., Komalavalli, C.: Recent advancements in the internet of things for the medical healthcare systems. Available at SSRN 4366731 (2023)

Investigating the Use of Utility Monitoring as a Means of Recognizing Activities of Daily Living (ADLs) to Enable Independent Living Among People Living with Dementia

Ciarán Nugent[1(✉)], Damon Berry[1], Jonathan Turner[1], Michael Wilson[2], Ann Marron[2], Julie Doyle[2], and Dympna O'Sullivan[1]

[1] Department of Computer Science, Technological University Dublin, Dublin, Ireland
{ciaran.nugent,damon.berry,jonathan.turner, dympna.osullivan}@tudublin.ie
[2] NetwellCASALA, Dundalk Institute of Technology, Dundalk, Ireland
{michael.wilson,julie.doyle}@dkit.ie, ann.marron@hse.ie

Abstract. Dementia can make it difficult for individuals to live independently, impacting their ability to carry out activities of daily living (ADLs). ADL data is frequently screened by clinicians using manual screening tools such as Katz' Index of Independence in Activities, Lawton Brody, and Barthel Index, to detect a degradation in the ability to complete ADLs. Identifying whether a person living with dementia (PLwD) can carry out an ADL can allow for early support to be provided.

This study explores the potential of utility monitoring to identify and monitor ADL achievement in PLwD. By leveraging Internet of Things (IoT) solutions and smart home sensors, including thermal sensors, door contacts, vibration sensors, wearable, motion sensors and smart plugs, utility monitoring is employed to capture ADL data. Through an open-source software framework, these sensors are integrated into a scalable and cost-effective architecture, enabling the real-time monitoring water and electricity usage. By analysing the data collected from these utilities, specific ADLs can be inferred, providing valuable insights into the daily routines and behaviours of PLwD.

This research contributes to the growing field of smart home sensor monitoring for ADL identification in dementia care. The results obtained from this study shed light on the feasibility and effectiveness of utility monitoring as a non-intrusive and scalable approach for supporting independent living in PLwD. The findings show potential areas for the development of innovative assistive technologies to enhance the quality of life for individuals with dementia and alleviate caregiver burden.

Keywords: Dementia · Activities of Daily Living · Utility Monitoring · Digital Toolkit · Independent Living

1 Introduction

Dementia is a term that is used for a range of conditions that cause damage to the brain. This damage can affect memory, other cognitive abilities, and behaviour that interferes significantly with a person's ability to maintain the ADLs. [1]. By 2050, it is expected that one new case of Alzheimer's Disease will develop every 33 s, resulting in almost 1 million new cases per year worldwide. People's ability to complete ADLs can decrease with Mild Cognitive Impairment and initial stages of Dementia. Research has indicated that the rate of decline in dementing illnesses can be slowed down by maintaining the ability to live independently.

The ability of older people to conduct ADLs, such as getting out of bed, toileting, bathing, dressing, grooming, and eating is frequently screened and assessed [2]. Measurement screenings and activities using psychometric instruments detect early-onset disabilities.

Screening tools that are used by clinicians and occupational therapists in the practice of identifying people's ability to complete ADLs include:

- Katz' Index of Independence in Activities of Daily Living (Basic ADLs (b-ADLs))

  – Bathing, dressing, toileting transferring, continence, and feeding. [3]

- Lawton Brody Instrumental Activities of Daily Living (Instrumental ADLs (I-ADLs)) [4]

  – Ability to Use Telephone, Shopping, Food Preparation, Housekeeping, Laundry, Mode of Transportation, Responsibility for Own Medication, Ability to Handle Finances.

- Barthel Index [5]

  – Bowels, Bladder, Grooming, Toilet Use, Feeding, Transfer, Mobility, Dressing, Stairs, Bathing.

Our research adopts a multidisciplinary approach to co-design innovative assistive technologies for PLwD. Our main focus lies in the creation of a comprehensive digital toolkit that facilitates the support and care of those with mild-to-moderate dementia, along with their informal caregivers.

This toolkit aims to enable the planning and monitoring of personalized care goals by incorporating targets derived from care plans, established models of daily activities, and activities that hold personal significance for both individuals with dementia and their caregivers. By integrating these elements, we strive to enhance the overall well-being and quality of life for PLwD, while also alleviating the burden on their caregivers.

Recent research has shown that IoT solutions can be utilised to identify ADLs. Smart home sensors, such as thermal, door contacts, vibration, wearable, and motion sensors are extensively used to identify ADLs. Sensor operations are utilised to infer whether an ADL is occurring. Expanding upon prior research in the realm of dementia sensing, this study leverages utility monitoring as a novel approach to track ADLs. Additionally, exploring the advantages of this method reveals several promising aspects, including simplified setup and maintenance due to reduced device requirements.

The architecture of the proposed framework will be designed around the following principles to enable the utilisation of low-cost off-the-shelf sensors and maintain control of data. The architecture has the following characteristics.

1. Open-Source Software
2. Local Network
3. Low Cost
4. Scalable

The rest of the paper is organized as follows: Sect. 2 provides a comprehensive literature review of relevant studies and prior research in the field. Section 3 offers an overview of the methods employed in this study, detailing the proposed architecture and energy monitoring approaches utilized.

The results obtained from the conducted research are presented in Sect. 4, showcasing the findings and their implications. Finally, Sect. 5 concludes the paper with a discussion, analysis of the results, and offers perspectives on utility monitoring to identify ADLs.

2 Literature Review

There is a significant amount of ongoing research using sensors to passively monitor and infer ADLs. The ability to capture ADLs is being completed in the laboratory and field. Many contemporary researchers utilise smart home sensors, mobile and wearable devices [6–11].

Several studies have been completed to monitor ADL achievement for PLwD with a focus on smart home sensors. Rawtaer et al. completed a cross-sectional study to establish the feasibility and acceptability of utilizing sensors in senior citizens' homes to detect changes in behaviours unobtrusively. Sensors such as smart plugs, a water usage sensor, passive infrared motion sensors, bed sensors, and a wearable activity band were deployed in the homes of community-dwelling senior citizens to monitor their behaviour patterns and detect potential signs of mild cognitive impairment. The water usage sensor was abandoned in this study as it was not deemed technically feasible [12]. Feng et al. focus on leveraging mobile data for activity recognition to enhance human well-being, using the data from mobile phone sensors [13]. Park et al. proposed the development of a self-organizing IoT device-based system for smart diagnosing assistance with ADLs. A pilot test was carried out in a hospital to recognise ADLs utilising smart home sensors such as acceleration, flame, temperature, and humidity. Appliance interaction was captured using General Purpose Input/Output (GPIO). Participants were instructed to complete ADLs via an electronic device [14]. Soma et al. monitored ADLs using an IOT system consisting of magnetic, motion, current transformer (CT), and tilt sensors [15].

In addition to smart home sensor studies, other completed studies have utilised mobile phone and wearable sensors. Mighali et al. presented an IOT system that can harness data from IOT sensors to capture positioning and motility data to detect behavioural deviations. Devices used in this study included Bluetooth Low Energy (BLE) beacons and a wearable hand band equipped with a triaxial accelerometer, gyroscope, magnetometer, and BLE transceiver. The beacons were placed strategically to provide proximity to key regions and periodically send out Unique Identification Codes to receiving devices, either the hand band or the smartphone, which also receives Received Signal Strength (RSS) values. These values are then used to indicate the relative positioning of the person indoors [16].

The majority of studies mentioned in the literature review are cross-sectional or feasibility studies. There is a need for more longitudinal studies that examine the long-term effectiveness and benefits of utility monitoring and smart home sensors in supporting independent living and tracking changes in ADL performance over time.

The accuracy and reliability of smart home sensors in inferring specific ADLs needs further validation. While these technologies hold promise, it is essential to evaluate their performance against established assessment tools and clinical observations to ensure their effectiveness in capturing ADLs accurately. One area which could augment the accuracy and reliability of monitoring ADL activity is utility monitoring such as work completed by Bilodeu et al. [17]. Sensors could be attached to the main incoming electrical cable to a home and also the main incoming water pipe. As electricity and water are used while completing many of the ADLs outlined in the screening tools mentioned before. The data gathered from these sensors could be used to increase accuracy when inferring ADL activity.

As the use of smart home sensors involves collecting personal data in private spaces, there is a need to address privacy concerns and ensure appropriate ethical practices. Research should focus on exploring strategies to safeguard sensitive data, obtain informed consent, and address any potential intrusiveness perceived by PLwD and other cohabitants.

The reviewed studies have predominantly focused on specific populations or settings, which may limit the generalizability of findings. Further research should involve diverse populations and consider cultural, social, and environmental factors that can influence ADLs and the acceptability of monitoring technologies across different contexts.

To ensure the successful adoption and long-term use of utility monitoring and smart home sensors, studies should prioritize user-centred design approaches. Engagement with PLwD, caregivers, and healthcare professionals in the development and evaluation of these technologies should enhance their acceptability, usability, and overall user satisfaction.

3 Proposed Methodology

This paper proposes monitoring energy usage to infer whether ADLs are being completed. Energy usage can identify a wide variety of ADLs including Food Preparation, Housekeeping, Laundry, and Bathing. Monitoring the electricity consumed on kitchen appliances can infer food preparation, the electricity consumed by a vacuum cleaner or dishwasher indicates housekeeping. A washing machine, tumble dryer or iron can indicate laundry. While the use of electrical devices: water heaters, power showers or immersion heaters can be used to infer bathing activity although monitoring water usage may be more appropriate.

Building on ADLs identified in previous papers [17] and from gaps identified in the literature review an architecture must be created to allow all types of in-home sensors from different manufacturers to be easily integrated. Initially, the architecture will be designed to capture electricity usage but it is envisaged that further smart home sensors will be required to demonstrate the accuracy of inferring ADL activity with and without utility monitoring. As data to be captured is personal in nature, data should be stored securely. From this, the architecture is built upon principles of Open-Source Software, Local Network, Low Cost, and Scalability, there rests a significant emphasis on ensuring a blend of versatility and security in deploying this system across diverse settings. Due the sensitive nature of collecting data in people's homes, particularly PLwD. Additional emphasis is given to ethical considerations.

3.1 Open-Source Software

Open-Source Software will be utilised as it allows for the use of sensors from different manufacturers and communication protocols to be managed with one system. This principle aligns with the study's objective by enabling a diverse array of sensors from various manufacturers to be integrated into the system, thereby enhancing the system's ability to monitor numerous ADL facets.

3.2 Local Network

All data will be stored within a local database on a local network with appropriate levels of security. As the data is very personal, the bulk of all data shall be stored within a local network with access limited to approved persons. Restricting data to a local network reduces the risk of personal data being exploited by third-party software platforms. This underscores a commitment to privacy and data security, vital given the sensitive nature of monitoring ADLs in vulnerable populations. This aligns with ethical considerations, ensuring that PLwD's daily activities are securely monitored and stored, protecting their dignity and privacy.

3.3 Low Cost

A low-cost approach not only ensures scalability but also aligns with an objective of inclusivity, ensuring that the benefits of ADL monitoring through smart technologies are accessible to a wide demographic. It addresses the financial challenges of implementing smart home solutions on a wider scale, thereby potentially democratizing access to supportive dementia care solutions and contributing to reducing disparities in care quality and availability.

3.4 Scalable

By prioritizing scalability, the architecture ensures that it can be adapted and expanded to accommodate advancements in sensor technology and emerging research on dementia and ADLs. Scalability implies the methodology can evolve to encapsulate more nuanced or additional ADLs in future, or to integrate with other smart home technologies, thereby ensuring the study remains relevant and adaptable to the dynamic needs and challenges of dementia care.

3.5 Ethical Considerations

Navigating the ethical landscape necessitates a blend of technological and humane strategies, particularly in managing sensitive data from PLwD. Initiating with informed consent, clear and accessible informational materials should be presented to PLwD and caregivers, followed by interactive sessions to assess understanding and acquire agreement. Stringent data security measures, involving robust encryption and access restrictions, safeguard participant privacy, while transparent documentation underscores data usage protocols. Upholding dignity involves respecting PLwD's physical and emotional boundaries and autonomy, facilitated through user-friendly interfaces. A continuous cycle of ethical evaluations and feedback mechanisms, coupled with defined withdrawal protocols, ensures sustained adherence to ethical practices throughout the study, weaving a framework that respects, protects, and empowers PLwD amidst technological interfacing and data management.

4 Sensor Framework

4.1 Architecture

Utilising the principles in the previous section, the architecture in Fig. 1 has been created. This paper is focused on using one type of sensor electricity monitoring, but the framework designed allows for many wireless sensors to be utilised to infer ADL activity

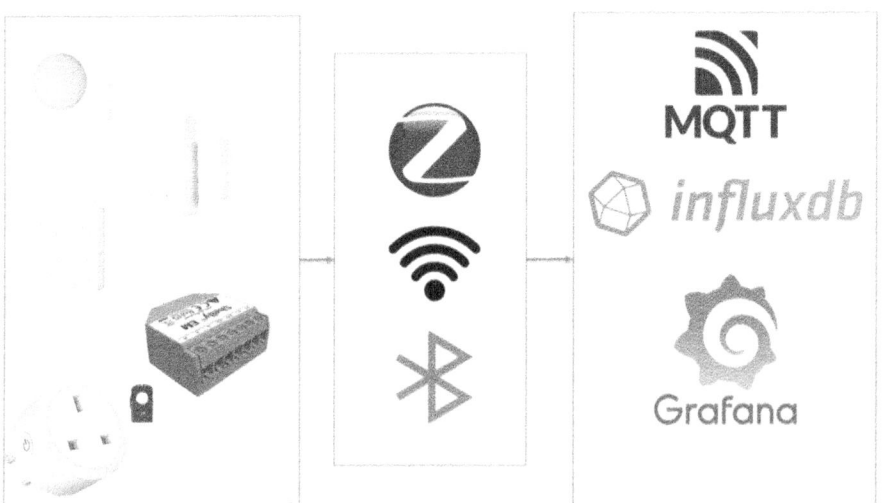

Fig. 1. Proposed SDC Architecture

such as thermal, door contacts, vibration, wearable, and motion sensors. From left to right, sensors communicate to a central device through various communication protocols. The packets of data pass through an MQTT broker. The data is homogenised and then populates a time-series database, InfluxDB. The data in the time-series database is analysed using rules set out to identify which ADL has been completed. An example of this could be seen using a toaster to prepare food: if the toaster has been switched on and consuming electricity (1,700 W - 2,200 W) for a period (2 min – 3 min). Then the basic and instrumental ADL activity of preparing food can be inferred. The information is then communicated to end-users via data visualisation tools.

4.2 Energy Monitoring

Energy usage can identify a wide variety of ADLs including Food Preparation, Housekeeping, Laundry, and Bathing. Monitoring the electricity consumed on kitchen appliances can infer food preparation, while the electricity consumed by a vacuum cleaner or dishwasher indicates housekeeping. Use of a washing machine, tumble dryer or iron can indicate laundry. In a similar way, the use of electrical devices: water heaters, power showers or immersion heaters can be used to infer bathing activity although monitoring water usage may be more appropriate.

The monitoring and testing took place in a household comprising four individuals; however, it should be noted that this home did not include a person with dementia. The electricity usage was monitored at the distribution board by installing a current transformer around the main incoming cable (refer to Fig. 2). Additionally, the monitoring encompassed the cooker circuit, as it is considered a fixed-wired appliance. To broaden the scope of monitoring, smart plugs were employed to track the electricity usage of specific devices, including a television, kettle, microwave, and toaster (as depicted in Fig. 3).

Figure 4 shows data recorded over a 24 h period in a home. The top graph shows the total electricity consumed. Devices such as a kettle, oven, microwave, and TV were captured using Wi-Fi CTs and smart plugs. The red box shows a kettle being used in the orange graph (spike of 2,500 W for 2 min) and an oven being used in the green graph (spike of 2200 W for 10 min). These two time series signals can be seen in the total electricity consumed by the house, blue graph as a spike which reaches circa 6,000 W but reduces to 3,000 W after a period of 2 min and further reduces to baseload 8 min later. The green box shows a 10,000 W signal for 5 min. This was an electric shower being used. The benefit of capturing data and main incoming data is that it is possible to capture all the electrical device/appliance usage like the electric show which would not be possible to connect to a smart plug due to the high load.

Appliance power consumption can be broken down into the following variables power used, real and reactive, and duration. All electrical current consumed in a home flows through the main incoming electrical power cable. Therefore, the powerline signature of every electrical appliance in a home can be monitored from the mains monitoring current transformer. The data will be analysed to identify which electrical appliance is being used. When the appliance usage is identified this can be used to infer what ADL is occurring at that time.

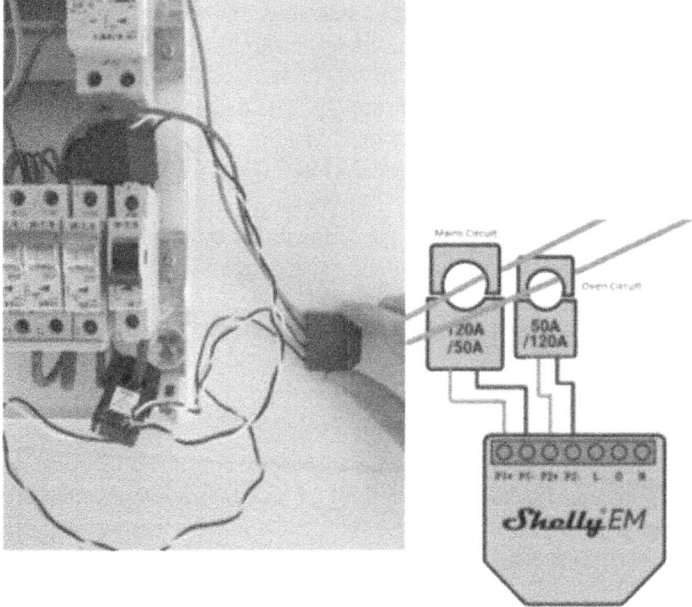

Fig. 2. Mains Power Monitoring

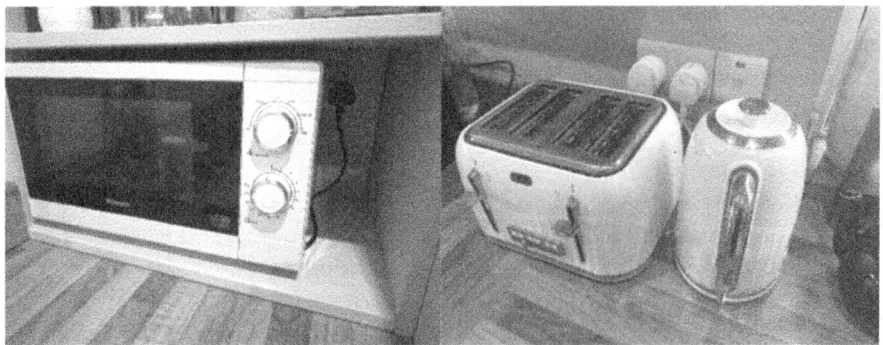

Fig. 3. Appliance Monitoring

To enhance the accuracy of our system that correlates ADL activity with energy usage, we propose the following multi-stage validation process. First, we have established an ADL Register by creating a comprehensive list of ADLs that can be inferred from energy consumption patterns. Next, we will subject the identified ADLs to controlled experiments in a laboratory setting. In this phase, each activity will be systematically performed and logged with precise timestamps to capture its unique energy signature. The testing will then transition to a real-world domestic environment, where participants will log their ADL activities using a dedicated smartphone application. This

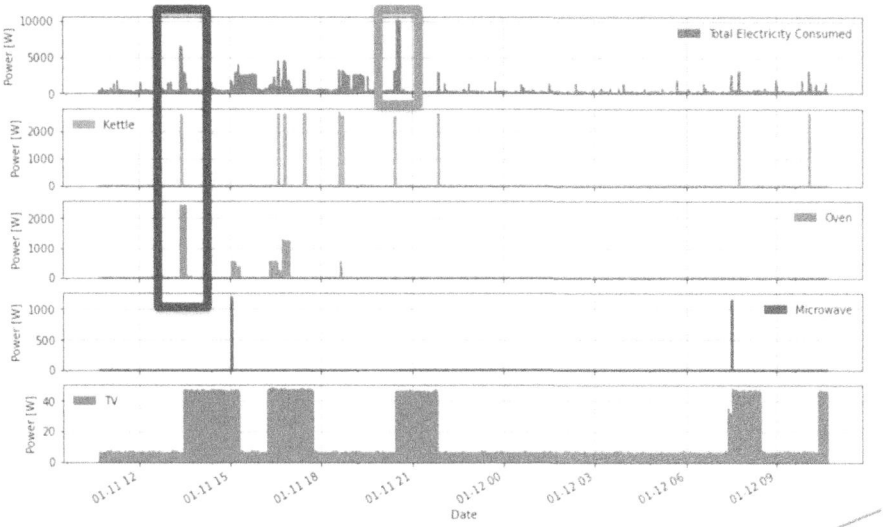

Fig. 4. Electrical Power Usage Main Incoming and Appliances

ensures we have an accurate record (the ground truth) against which energy consumption inferences can be compared. Lastly, we will extend the system's testing to homes of PLwD to assess its practicality, accuracy, and usability in real-world scenarios tailored to this demographic.

5 Conclusion

By observing the activities of ADLs for PLwD, we can empower them to maintain an independent lifestyle within the familiar comforts of their own home. This paper proposes the implementation of a sensor framework that incorporates smart home in-home sensors to identify ADLs and facilitate subsequent analysis. The framework combines the information from inexpensive off-the-shelf smart home devices with utility energy monitoring as a potential application to identify ADL activities for PLwD. This paper introduces a proposed implementation of a sensor framework that incorporates smart home in-home sensors to identify ADLs and facilitate subsequent analysis. As part of our research, we will actively engage dementia specialists, groups, and PLwD to gather valuable insights into the suitability of using sensors for ADL monitoring. We acknowledge that living with smart home sensors in a home may raise concerns about intrusion, and we will actively seek feedback from both PLwD and other cohabitants to address any concerns. Living with smart home sensors in a home can feel intrusive to the people living in the residence. Feedback on concerns will be sought from both the person living with Dementia/MCI and any other cohabitants.

To begin, we will identify commercially available sensors, taking into consideration factors such as communication protocol, power usage, range, and cost. This critical information will guide us in selecting appropriate sensors for our framework. We will then create a robust communication system capable of efficiently collecting data from sensors that use different communication protocols. As data packets from different manufacturers may have varying formats, we will homogenize the data and pass it into a structured time series database.

Next, we will determine which ADLs can be effectively monitored using utility sensors. We will create a comprehensive register of ADLs and utilize sensors to track these specific activities. The collected data will be carefully analysed to identify when a selected ADL has occurred. To ensure usability for end users, the data will be appropriately aggregated to facilitate interpretation. A register of ADLs will be created, and sensors can be used to monitor these ADLs. The data will be analysed to identify a selected ADL has occurred. The data should be aggregated to allow for interpretation of end users.

References

1. World Health Organization, "Dementia: Fact sheet," World Health Organization (2017). https://www.who.int/news-room/fact-sheets/detail/dementia. Accessed 12 Jan 2022
2. Hopman-Rock, M., van Hirtum, H., de Vreede, P., Freiberger, E.: Activities of daily living in older community-dwelling persons: a systematic review of psychometric properties of instruments. Aging Clin. Exp. Res. **31**(7), 917–925 (2018)
3. Katz, S.F.A.B., Moskowitz, R.W., Jackson, B.A., Jaffe, M.W.: Studies of illness in the aged: the index of ADL: a standardized measure of biological and psychosocial function. J. Am. Med. Assoc. **185**(12), 914–919 (1963)
4. Assessment of older people: Self-maintaining and instrumental activities of daily living. The Gerontologist **9**(3), 179–186 (1969)
5. Barthel, D., Mahoney, F.: Functional evaluation: the barthel index: a simple index of independence useful in scoring improvement in the rehabilitation of the chronically ill. Md. State Med. J. **14**, 61–65 (1965)
6. Tewell, J., O'Sullivan, D., Maiden, N., Lockerbie, J., Stumpf, S.: Monitoring meaningful activities using small low-cost devices in a smart home. Pers. Ubiquit. Comput. **23**(2), 339–357 (2019)
7. Tan, H.-X., Tan, H.-P.: Early detection of mild cognitive impairment in elderly through IOT: Preliminary findings. In: 2018 IEEE 4th World Forum on Internet of Things (WF-IoT) (2018)
8. Enshaeifar, S. et al.: Health Management and pattern analysis of daily living activities of people with dementia using in-home sensors and Machine Learning Techniques. PLOS ONE **13**(5) (2018)
9. Sokullu, R., Akkaş, M., Demir, E.: IOT supported smart home for the elderly. Internet of Things **11**, 100239 (2020)
10. Takahashi, Y., Nishida, Y., Kitamura, K., Mizoguchi, H.: Handrail IOT sensor for precision healthcare of elderly people in Smart Homes. In: 2017 IEEE International Symposium on Robotics and Intelligent Sensors (IRIS) (2017)
11. Klavestad, S., Assres, G., Fagernes, S., Grønli, T.-M.: Monitoring activities of daily living using UWB radar technology: a contactless approach. IoT **1**(2), 320–336 (2020)
12. Rawtaer, I., et al.: Early detection of mild cognitive impairment with in-home sensors to monitor behavior patterns in community-dwelling senior citizens in Singapore: cross-sectional feasibility study. J. Medical Internet Res. **22**(5) (2020)
13. Feng, Y., Chang, C., Ming, H.: Engaging mobile data to improve human well-being: the ADL recognition approach. IT Professional, p. 1 (2017)

14. Park, Y.J., Jung, S.Y., Son, T.Y., Kang, S.J.: Self-organizing IOT device-based smart diagnosing assistance system for activities of daily living. Sensors **21**(3), 785 (2021)
15. Soma, T., Lawanont, W., Yokemura, T., Inoue, M.: Monitoring system for detecting decrease of living motivation based on change in activities of daily living. In: 2020 IEEE International Conference on Consumer Electronics (ICCE), Las Vegas (2020)
16. Mighali, V., Patrono, L., Stefanizzi, M.L., Rodrigues, J.J., Solic, P.: A smart remote elderly monitoring system based on IOT Technologies. In: 2017 Ninth International Conference on Ubiquitous and Future Networks (ICUFN) (2017)
17. Bilodeau, J.-S., Fortin-Simard, D., Gaboury, S., Bouchard, B., Bouzouane, A.: Assistance in smart homes: Combining passive RFID localization and load signatures of electrical devices. In: IEEE International Conference on Bioinformatics and Biomedicine (BIBM), Belfast (2014)
18. Turner, J., et al.: A goal-driven framework for individualised self-care for early-stage dementia. International Journal on Advances in Life Sciences **14**(1) (2022)

Enhancing Transparency and Trustworthiness of Healthcare IoT Data with AWS: A Proposed Model

Zahra Ali[1], Abdul Ahad[2,3(✉)], Filipe Madeira[4(✉)], and Ibraheem Shayea[3]

[1] Department of Computer Science, University of Management and Technology, Sialkot 51040, Pakistan
zahra.ali@skt.umt.edu.pk
[2] School of Software, Northwestern Polytechnical University, Xian, Shaanxi, People's Republic of China
ahad9388@gmail.com
[3] Department of Electronics and Communication Engineering, Istanbul Technical University (ITU), 34467 Istanbul, Turkey
shayea@itu.edu.tr
[4] Department of Informatics and Quantitative Methods, Research Center for Arts and Communication (CIAC)/Pole of Digital Literacy and Social Inclusion, Polytechnic Institute of Santarem, Street, 2001-904 Santarem, Portugal
filipe.madeira@esg.ipsantarem.pt

Abstract. The growing adoption of healthcare Internet of Things (IoT) devices has led to an exponential increase in the generation and sharing of sensitive patient data. However, ensuring transparency and trustworthiness of healthcare IoT data remains a critical concern. This research paper presents a novel approach to address these challenges by proposing a model that leverages Amazon Web Services (AWS). The model integrates various AWS services to establish secure data storage, encryption, access controls, audit logs, compliance, and data analytics, all while prioritizing data privacy through anonymization techniques. A comprehensive literature review underscores the significance of transparency and trust in healthcare IoT data, highlighting the need for robust mechanisms. The model encompasses AWS S3 and Glacier for encrypted, scalable data storage, AWS KMS for data encryption and key management, AWS IAM for access controls, and AWS CloudTrail and CloudWatch for monitoring and auditing. Additionally, AWS Lambda and Amazon Redshift are employed for data analytics. The paper outlines implementation and deployment considerations, including integration with existing healthcare IoT infrastructure, offering practical steps for implementation. Through case studies and comparative analysis, the advantages of the proposed model are demonstrated. The evaluation metrics and methods outlined enable the assessment of transparency and trustworthiness of healthcare IoT data facilitated by the proposed model. This research contributes a valuable framework for healthcare IoT stakeholders to enhance transparency and trustworthiness in their data management utilizing AWS services, while

---

Z. Ali and I. Shayea—Contributing authors.

also identifying future research directions for continuous improvement in healthcare IoT data governance and trust-building mechanisms.

Keywords: Healthcare IoT · Data privacy · Amazon Web service AWS · Anonymization techniques

1 Introduction

The rapid advancement and widespread adoption of healthcare Internet of Things (IoT) devices have transformed the landscape of modern healthcare. These devices, ranging from wearable sensors to connected medical equipment, have the potential to revolutionize patient care, improve diagnostics, and enhance overall healthcare outcomes. However, along with the numerous benefits that healthcare IoT brings, there are significant concerns regarding the transparency and trustworthiness of the data generated and shared by these devices [1].

The need for transparency and trust in healthcare IoT data arises from the sensitive nature of patient information and the critical decisions that healthcare professionals make based on this data [2]. Patients and stakeholders must have confidence in the integrity, security, and privacy of the healthcare IoT ecosystem. Without adequate measures to ensure transparency and trust, users may hesitate to embrace healthcare IoT solutions, leading to limited adoption and compromised healthcare delivery [3].

This research paper aims to address the pressing challenge of enhancing transparency and trustworthiness in healthcare IoT data by proposing a novel model that leverages Amazon Web Services (AWS) - a leading cloud computing platform. By combining various AWS services specifically designed for data security, privacy, and analytics, the proposed model offers a comprehensive framework to establish transparency and build trust in healthcare IoT environments.

Through an extensive review of existing literature, this paper underscores the significance of transparency and trust in healthcare IoT data, exploring the current gaps in research and practice. By identifying the limitations of existing approaches, we present a novel model that harnesses the capabilities of AWS services to overcome these challenges and enhance the transparency and trustworthiness of healthcare IoT data.

The model encompasses a range of AWS services tailored to meet the unique demands of healthcare IoT, including secure data storage, robust data encryption, fine-grained access controls, comprehensive audit logs, compliance management, and advanced data analytics while preserving patient privacy through anonymization techniques. By utilizing these AWS services, our proposed model offers a comprehensive and practical solution to establish transparency and trust, paving the way for secure and effective healthcare IoT implementations.

In the subsequent sections of this paper, we will delve into the details of our proposed model, discussing the individual components, practical implementation considerations, case studies showcasing its effectiveness, and evaluation metrics to assess the transparency and trustworthiness of healthcare IoT data facilitated by the model. By presenting this research, we aim to provide valuable insights and actionable recommendations for healthcare IoT stakeholders to strengthen transparency and trust in their data management practices.

Overall, this research contributes to the evolving field of healthcare IoT by offering a practical and scalable framework that leverages AWS services, thereby enabling stakeholders to enhance transparency and trustworthiness in healthcare IoT data. By fostering confidence among users, healthcare IoT can unlock its full potential, revolutionizing healthcare delivery and improving patient outcomes.

2 Literature Review

In papers [4–6], challenges of clustering, routing, privacy and security are discussed for smart heatlhcare. It highlights the challenges for secure medical data transmission in remote patient monitoring. Healthcare providers are primarily motivated by the need to secure protected health information (PHI), which makes healthcare data a valuable target for hackers. Blockchain technology is the ideal solution for the healthcare system and might solve these problems because data in blocks cannot be deleted or changed. Hence cloud-based blockchain services are an ideal solution for protecting patients' records in health care. Moreover, the paper [7], provided an overview of IoT applications, advantages, and potential hazards, the article "IoT Privacy and Security: Challenges and Solutions" suggests a new IoT layered architecture. The study also builds new security schemes and analyses existing ones, offering suggestions to reduce risks and address potential security flaws. The need for regulatory bodies to enforce rules, for end users and entities to be educated, and for IoT stakeholders to create and implement suitable security and privacy safeguards are some of the issues that will arise in the future. The paper [8], highlights the importance of the Internet of Things (IoT) in this context and how it has become a hot research topic in recent years. In the future, a fog computing environment can be added to the existing infrastructure to increase the overall performance of the proposed model. In the paper [9], the authors proposed a smart option based on IoT and ML to improve standards of living and prove crucial in saving human lives. Cloud-oriented services are best for handling this kind of scenario. In the paper [10], the authors proposed a chatbot, that acts as a pregnancy companion to the women to answer their immediate questions. But the proposed model has many privacy concerns e.g. access control issues. These issues need to be addressed in the future using cloud computing services e.e IAM service in Amazon. In the paper [11], the authors discuss in detail how AWS can provide the best services in a healthcare environment. But it is case studies that how with different environments and requirements AWS services are suitable in the healthcare environment. In the paper [12], the authors proposed smart and economic telemedicine solutions using deep reinforcement learning. It has improved the overall system performance. In the future, the patient dataset can be analyzed with other deep learning algorithms to improve the overall performance of telemedicine systems.

In [13] a framework is proposed that is handling the healthcare data using AWS services. However, the proposed work is lacking with some unauthorized access of data, that can be handled in the AWS environment by adding some more access control to data to prevent it from unauthorized access. Hence there is a need to implement cloud-based services in the healthcare environment to increase its overall performance.

3 Proposed Model: Transparency and Trust-Enhancing Framework Using AWS Services

The proposed model aims to establish transparency and enhance trustworthiness in healthcare IoT data by leveraging a carefully designed framework that harnesses the capabilities of Amazon Web Services (AWS). By integrating various AWS services, the model provides a robust and comprehensive solution to address the challenges associated with transparency and trust in healthcare IoT environments as shown in Fig. 1. Secure Data Storage: The foundation of the proposed framework lies in secure data storage, achieved through AWS S3 (Simple Storage Service) and AWS Glacier. These services offer encrypted and scalable storage solutions, ensuring the confidentiality and integrity of healthcare IoT data. By leveraging AWS's advanced security features, such as server-side encryption and access controls, the proposed model establishes a secure foundation for storing sensitive patient information.

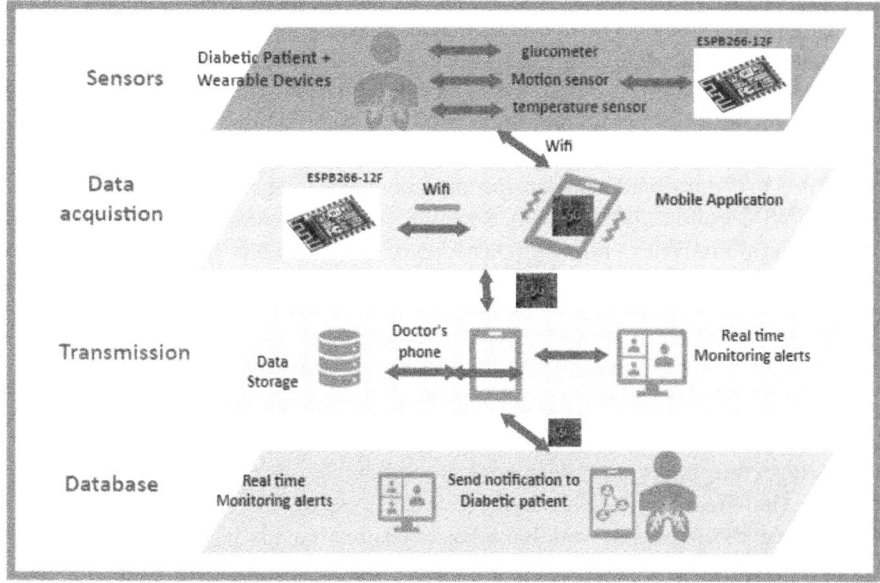

Fig. 1. Proposed Solution for enhancing transparency and trust in healthcare-IoT

Data Encryption: To further bolster data security, the proposed model incorporates AWS Key Management Service (KMS) for data encryption and key management. With KMS, healthcare IoT data can be encrypted at rest and in transit, mitigating the risk of unauthorized access or data breaches. By managing encryption keys centrally and enforcing strong encryption practices, the proposed model ensures that healthcare IoT data remains protected throughout its lifecycle.

Access Controls and Identity Management: Ensuring the appropriate access controls and identity management is crucial for maintaining the trustworthiness of healthcare IoT data. The proposed model leverages AWS Identity and Access Management (IAM) to enforce fine-grained access policies and user authentication. By assigning unique credentials and access permissions to authorized individuals or entities, the model safeguards against unauthorized data access and unauthorized modifications.

Audit Logs and Monitoring: Transparency is fostered through comprehensive audit logs and monitoring mechanisms. The proposed model incorporates AWS CloudTrail and AWS CloudWatch to enable detailed monitoring, logging, and auditing of healthcare IoT data access and usage. These services provide visibility into data modifications, access attempts, and system activities, enhancing transparency and accountability while enabling prompt identification of any suspicious or unauthorized activities.

Compliance and Privacy: Adhering to industry regulations and privacy requirements is critical in healthcare IoT environments. The proposed model incorporates AWS services such as AWS Artifact and AWS Control Tower to facilitate compliance management. These services offer a robust framework for maintaining and demonstrating compliance with regulations such as the Health Insurance Portability and Accountability Act (HIPAA) and the General Data Protection Regulation (GDPR). By adhering to these standards, the proposed model enhances trust in the handling of healthcare IoT data.

Data Analytics and Anonymization: To extract meaningful insights from healthcare IoT data while preserving patient privacy, the proposed model integrates AWS Lambda and Amazon Redshift. These services enable efficient and scalable data analytics, allowing healthcare professionals and researchers to derive valuable insights from the data. Additionally, the proposed model emphasizes the use of anonymization techniques to protect patient identities during data analysis, ensuring privacy while maintaining the usefulness of the data.

By combining these AWS services, the proposed model establishes a comprehensive framework that enhances transparency and trustworthiness in healthcare IoT data. The model addresses key aspects of data security, access controls, monitoring, compliance, and data analytics, all while prioritizing patient privacy. Through the effective utilization of AWS services, healthcare IoT stakeholders can leverage a trusted and scalable infrastructure that instills confidence among users and facilitates the responsible utilization of healthcare IoT data.

In the subsequent sections of this research paper, we will discuss the implementation and deployment considerations of the proposed model, including practical steps for integrating the framework into existing healthcare IoT infrastructures. We will also present case studies and comparative analyses to demonstrate the advantages and effectiveness of the proposed model in enhancing transparency and trustworthiness in healthcare IoT environments.

3.1 Implementation

Implementing the proposed transparency and trust-enhancing framework using AWS services requires careful planning and consideration of various factors. This subsection discusses key implementation considerations to ensure the successful deployment of the model in healthcare IoT environments.

Infrastructure Integration: Integrating the proposed framework with existing healthcare IoT infrastructure is a crucial step. It involves assessing the compatibility and requirements of the AWS services with the existing systems, devices, and data workflows. This integration may require modifications or extensions to the infrastructure to establish seamless communication and data exchange between the healthcare IoT devices and the AWS services.

Security and Privacy: As healthcare IoT deals with sensitive patient data, security, and privacy must be prioritized during implementation. It is essential to configure AWS services, such as AWS S3, Glacier, and KMS, with strong encryption protocols and access controls to safeguard the data. Additionally, adherence to best practices for secure data transmission, such as utilizing secure protocols like HTTPS and ensuring secure device authentication, must be considered to prevent unauthorized access or data breaches.

Scalability and Performance: Healthcare IoT generates a massive volume of data, and the proposed model should be scalable to handle increasing data volumes efficiently. AWS services like S3 and Redshift provide scalability options, enabling the infrastructure to accommodate growing data demands. Performance considerations, such as selecting appropriate AWS service configurations and optimizing data processing workflows, should be taken into account to ensure the efficient processing and analysis of healthcare IoT data.

Training and User Adoption: A successful implementation relies on the proper training and adoption of the proposed model by healthcare professionals and stakeholders. It is important to provide comprehensive training programs and documentation to familiarize users with the AWS services and the proposed framework. This will ensure that users can effectively utilize the system, follow data privacy guidelines, and make informed decisions based on transparent and trustworthy healthcare IoT data.

Compliance and Regulations: Compliance with industry regulations, such as HIPAA and GDPR, is critical in healthcare IoT environments. During implementation, it is crucial to configure AWS services according to the relevant compliance requirements. AWS Artifact and AWS Control Tower can be leveraged to streamline compliance management and ensure adherence to regulatory standards. Regular audits and assessments should be conducted to verify compliance and maintain data integrity.

Continuous Monitoring and Evaluation: Once the proposed framework is implemented, continuous monitoring and evaluation are essential to ensure its effectiveness and address any potential issues. AWS CloudTrail and CloudWatch should be configured to provide real-time monitoring of system activities and generate alerts for suspicious events. Regular evaluations of system performance, data integrity, and user feedback will help identify areas for improvement and fine-tune of the implemented framework.

By considering these implementation considerations, healthcare IoT stakeholders can effectively deploy the proposed transparency and trust-enhancing framework using AWS services. Adapting the infrastructure, ensuring security and privacy, scalability, user training, compliance management, and continuous monitoring are crucial aspects that contribute to a successful implementation, fostering transparency and trust in healthcare IoT data.

3.2 Comparative Analysis

In this section, we present a comparative analysis of cloud services provided by AWS, GCP, and Azure for enhancing the transparency and trustworthiness of healthcare IoT data. The analysis is based on key parameters, including data privacy and security, audit and compliance features, data governance and consent management, blockchain integration, data access, and control, data provenance and audibility, interoperability and standards support, transparency and explainability of AI/ML models, and vendor lock-in. The comparison aims to provide insights into the strengths and weaknesses of each cloud service provider in addressing the specific requirements of the healthcare industry as shown in Table 1.

In this comparison Table 1, we have assessed various parameters to compare AWS, GCP, and Azure in the context of enhancing the transparency and trustworthiness of healthcare IoT data. The table provides a visual representation of the features and capabilities of each cloud provider's specific services.

When it comes to data privacy and security, all three providers (AWS, GCP, and Azure) excel in implementing strong security measures, encryption, and access controls, while also meeting compliance certifications. Audit and compliance features are available across the board, allowing organizations to maintain detailed audit logs and utilize compliance reporting tools.

In terms of data governance and consent management, all three providers offer solutions like AWS Identity and Access Management (IAM) and AWS Key Management Service (KMS) to ensure proper data governance and access control. However, blockchain integration, data provenance, and auditability features are currently not supported by any of the mentioned services.

Interoperability and standards support, especially for healthcare IoT data, are more prominent in AWS compared to GCP and Azure. AWS provides support for HL7 and FHIR interoperability standards. On the other hand, GCP and Azure have limited support in this area.

Transparency and explainability of AI/ML models are currently lacking in all the mentioned services, including AWS, GCP, and Azure. These providers have yet to offer comprehensive solutions in this regard.

Table 1. Comparison of Cloud Service Providers

Parameters	Cloud Service Providers						
	AWS CloudTrail	AWS CloudWatch	AWS S3	AWS Glacier	AWS Lambda	Redshift	AWS KMS
Data Privacy and Security	✔	✔	✔	✔	✔	✔	✔
Audit and Compliance Features	✔	✔	✔	✔	✔	✔	✔
Data Governance and Consent Management	✔	✔	✔	✔	✔	✔	✔
Blockchain Integration	X	X	X	X	X	X	X
Data Access and Control	✔	✔	✔	✔	✔	✔	✔
Data Provenance and Auditability	✔	✔	X	X	X	X	X
Interoperability and Standards Support	✔	X	X	X	X	X	X
Transparency and Explainability of AI/ML Models	X	X	X	X	X	X	X
Vendor Lock-in	X	X	X	X	X	X	X

Considering the parameter of vendor lock-in, it is worth noting that all three cloud providers require some effort if switching from one to another. However, they do provide tools and services to facilitate migration and avoid excessive vendor lock-in.

Overall, based on the comparison table, AWS demonstrates strength in several areas such as data privacy and security, audit and compliance features, data governance and consent management, and interoperability standards support. However, the choice of the best cloud provider ultimately depends on specific healthcare IoT requirements, budget, scalability needs, and existing infrastructure of the organization.

Further, there is another comparison is done based on AWS service with GCP equivalent services to analyze which service provider is best fit for the trusted healthcare environment as shown in Table 2. When comparing the services provided by Google Cloud Platform (GCP) and Amazon Web Services (AWS) for healthcare IoT scenarios, several parameters were considered. Let's explore the key aspects of these services:

Data Privacy and Security: Both GCP and AWS offer robust measures to ensure data privacy and security. They provide encryption options, access controls, and compliance certifications to safeguard healthcare IoT data.

Audit and Compliance Features: GCP and AWS services include features for auditing and compliance, allowing healthcare organizations to meet regulatory requirements. They offer comprehensive logging, monitoring, and reporting capabilities.

Data Governance and Consent Management: Both platforms excel in data governance and consent management. GCP and AWS provide tools and frameworks to manage data access, consent, and governance policies, enabling organizations to maintain control over their healthcare IoT data.

Blockchain Integration: Unfortunately, neither GCP nor AWS currently offers native support for blockchain integration. If blockchain integration is a crucial requirement, alternative solutions or third-party services may need to be considered.

Data Access and Control: GCP and AWS provide robust mechanisms for managing data access and control. They offer fine-grained access controls, identity and access management, and data sharing options to ensure authorized access to healthcare IoT data.

Data Provenance and Auditability: While GCP excels in data provenance and auditability, offering detailed tracking and tracing of data lineage, AWS services have limited capabilities in this area. GCP's features enable organizations to establish clear data trails and maintain an audit history for compliance purposes.

Scalability: Both GCP and AWS services are highly scalable, allowing healthcare IoT applications to handle varying workloads and accommodate growing data volumes. They provide auto-scaling capabilities, flexible storage options, and robust infrastructure to meet scalability needs.

Cost-effectiveness: GCP and AWS offer cost-effective solutions, but pricing structures may vary based on service usage, storage requirements, and data transfer. It's important to carefully analyze the specific needs and pricing models to determine the most cost-effective option for healthcare IoT applications.

Overall, GCP and AWS provide competitive services for enhancing the transparency and trustworthiness of healthcare IoT data. While GCP offers strong features in data provenance and audibility, both platforms excel in areas such as data privacy, security, compliance, and scalability. Depending on the specific requirements, budget, scalability needs, and existing infrastructure of healthcare organizations, a careful evaluation should be conducted to determine the best-fit cloud provider for their healthcare IoT deployments.

The Table 2 provides a comparative analysis of AWS and Azure services in terms of enhancing the transparency and trustworthiness of healthcare IoT data.

In terms of data privacy, both AWS and Azure offer robust features to ensure the security and confidentiality of healthcare IoT data, indicated by the checkmarks in the respective columns. They also excel in audit and compliance, providing comprehensive tools to monitor and enforce regulatory requirements.

When it comes to data governance, AWS demonstrates strength across all services, whereas Azure lacks support for data governance features. However, Azure compensates with its strong offering in Azure Monitor, Azure Storage, and Azure Data Lake, which align well with the requirements of healthcare IoT data management.

Table 2. Comparison of Cloud Service Providers

Parameters	Cloud Service Providers						
	GCP Cloud Audit Logs	GCP Stackdriver	GCP Cloud Storage	GCP Coldline Storage	GCP Cloud Functions	GCP BigQuery	GCP Key Management Service (KMS)
Data Privacy and Security	✔	✔	✔	✔	✔	✔	✔
Audit and Compliance Features	✔	✔	✔	✔	✔	✔	✔
Data Governance and Consent Management	✔	✔	✔	✔	✔	✔	✔
Blockchain Integration	X	X	X	X	X	X	X
Data Access and Control	✔	✔	✔	✔	✔	✔	✔
Data Provenance and Auditability	✔	✔	X	X	X	X	X
Interoperability and Standards Support	✔	X	X	X	X	X	X
Transparency and Explainability of AI/ML Models	X	X	X	X	X	X	X
Vendor Lock-in	X	X	X	X	X	X	X

AWS outperforms Azure in data access control, offering a wide range of mechanisms to enforce fine-grained access policies. Additionally, AWS services such as AWS CloudTrail and AWS CloudWatch provide detailed logs and monitoring capabilities to track data access and usage.

While both cloud providers lack blockchain integration, which could enhance the immutability and transparency of healthcare IoT data, they compensate with other robust security features.

In terms of data provenance and interoperability, both AWS and Azure have limited support, as indicated by the absence of checkmarks in those columns.

Overall, AWS demonstrates a stronger presence in the healthcare IoT space, with its comprehensive suite of services like AWS S3, AWS Lambda, and Redshift that cater to the specific needs of healthcare data management. However, Azure offers a competitive alternative, particularly in areas such as Azure Monitor, Azure Storage, and Azure Data Lake.

Ultimately, the choice between AWS and Azure will depend on the specific requirements, budget, and existing infrastructure of healthcare organizations seeking to enhance the transparency and trustworthiness of their IoT data.

In summary, when comparing AWS, GCP, and Azure services for healthcare IoT, each provider brings its own strengths and considerations to the Table 3. AWS shines with its comprehensive suite of services, covering all aspects of

Table 3. Comparison of Azure Services

Parameters	Azure Sentinel	Azure Monitor	Azure Blob Storage	Azure Archive Storage	Azure Functions	Azure Synapse Analytics	Azure Key Vault
Data Privacy and Security	✓	✓	✓	✓	✓	✓	✓
Audit and Compliance Features	✓	✓	✓	✓	✓	✓	✓
Data Governance	✓	✓	✓	✓	✓	✓	✓
Blockchain Integration	×	×	×	×	×	×	×
Data Access and Control	✓	✓	✓	✓	✓	✓	✓
Data Provenance and Auditability	✓	✓	×	×	×	×	×
Interoperability and Standards	✓	×	✓	✓	×	✓	✓
Transparency and Explainability of AI/ML Models	×	×	×	×	×	×	×
Vendor Lock-in	✓	✓	✓	✓	✓	✓	✓

healthcare data management. With services like AWS CloudTrail, AWS CloudWatch, AWS S3, AWS Glacier, AWS Lambda, Redshift, and AWS KMS, AWS offers robust features for data privacy, compliance, access control, and data interoperability.

GCP holds its ground with offerings such as Cloud Audit Logs, Stackdriver Monitoring, Cloud Storage, Cloud Functions, BigQuery, and Cloud Key Management Services, providing solid capabilities for healthcare IoT data management. Azure, too, presents viable alternatives with Azure Monitor, Azure Storage, Azure Functions, Azure Data Lake Storage, Azure SQL Data Warehouse, and Azure Key Vault. While GCP and Azure have their strengths in specific areas, AWS emerges as the clear leader in terms of the breadth and depth of services available. Its comprehensive portfolio covers a wide range of healthcare IoT requirements. When making a decision, healthcare organizations should consider their specific needs, budget, scalability requirements, and existing infrastructure. By carefully evaluating these factors and taking into account the strengths of each cloud provider, organizations can make an informed choice that aligns with their goals of enhancing the transparency and trustworthiness of healthcare IoT data.

3.3 Conclusion

Based on our findings, AWS emerges as the leading cloud provider in terms of the breadth and depth of services offered. With offerings such as AWS CloudTrail, AWS CloudWatch, AWS S3, AWS Glacier, AWS Lambda, Redshift, and

AWS KMS, AWS provides a robust and comprehensive suite of services that cover various aspects of healthcare IoT data management. These services contribute to enhancing transparency, ensuring data security, and maintaining the trustworthiness of healthcare IoT data. While GCP and Azure also offer competitive services in specific areas, AWS stands out as the most suitable choice for healthcare organizations looking to enhance transparency and trustworthiness in their IoT data infrastructure.

3.4 Future Work

There are many aspects that should be considered in the future. Firstly, conducting in-depth case studies and practical implementations of the proposed model in real-world healthcare IoT environments would provide valuable insights into its effectiveness and scalability. Additionally, exploring the integration of emerging technologies such as blockchain and federated learning with cloud services could further enhance the transparency and security of healthcare IoT data. Overall, our research establishes AWS as a strong candidate for healthcare IoT data management, and the proposed model offers a foundation for organizations to enhance transparency and trustworthiness in their healthcare IoT infrastructure. In the future, there is a need to explore this field further to contribute to healthcare systems and the secure and ethical use of IoT data.

Acknowledgment. This work is funded by national funds through FCT - Foundation for Science and Technology, I.P., under project UIDP/04019/2020.

References

1. Ahad, A., et al.: A comprehensive review on 5G-based smart healthcare network security: taxonomy, issues, solutions and future research directions, *Array*, p. 100290 (2023)
2. Ahmed, M., Zubair, S.: Explainable artificial intelligence in sustainable smart healthcare. In: Ahmed, M., Islam, S.R., Anwar, A., Moustafa, N., Pathan, AS.K. (eds.) Explainable Artificial Intelligence for Cyber Security. SCI, vol. 1025, pp. 265–280. Springer, Cham (2022). https://doi.org/10.1007/978-3-030-96630-0_12
3. Ahad, A., Tahir, M.: Perspective-6G and IoT for intelligent healthcare: challenges and future research directions. ECS Sens. Plus **2**(1), 011601 (2023)
4. Tawalbeh, L., Muheidat, F., Tawalbeh, M., Quwaider, M.: IoT privacy and security: challenges and solutions. Appl. Sci. **10**(12), 4102 (2020)
5. Ahad, A., Tahir, M., Sheikh, M.A.S., Hassan, N., Ahmed, K.I., Mughees, A.: A game theory based clustering scheme (GCS) for 5G-based smart healthcare. In: 2020 IEEE 5th International Symposium on Telecommunication Technologies (ISTT), pp. 157–161. IEEE (2020)
6. Ahad, A., Tahir, M., Sheikh, M.A.S., Mughees, A., Ahmed, K.I.: Optimal route selection in 5G-based smart health-care network: a reinforcement learning approach. In: 2021 26th IEEE Asia-Pacific Conference on Communications (APCC), pp. 248–253. IEEE (2021)

7. Dwivedi, A.D., Srivastava, G., Dhar, S., Singh, R.: A decentralized privacy-preserving healthcare blockchain for IoT. Sensors **19**(2), 326 (2019)
8. Tawalbeh, M., Quwaider, M., Lo'ai, A.T.: Authorization model for IoT healthcare systems: case study. In: 2020 11th International Conference on Information and Communication Systems (ICICS), pp. 337–342. IEEE (2020)
9. Ashfaq, Z., et al.: Embedded AI-based Digi-healthcare. Appl. Sci. **12**(1), 519 (2022)
10. Sadavarte, S.S., Bodanese, E.: Pregnancy companion chatbot using Alexa and Amazon web services. In: 2019 IEEE Pune Section International Conference (PuneCon), pp. 1–5. IEEE (2019)
11. Dudhe, P., Kadam, N., Hushangabade, R., Deshmukh, M.: Internet of things (IoT): an overview and its applications. In: 2017 International Conference on Energy, Communication, Data Analytics and Soft Computing (ICECDS), pp. 2650–2653. IEEE (2017)
12. Jagannath, D.J., Dolly, R.J., Let, G.S., Peter, J.D.: An IoT enabled smart healthcare system using deep reinforcement learning. Concurr. Comput. Pract. Exper. **34**(28), e7403 (2022)
13. Rahamathulla, M.P., et al.: Cloud-based healthcare data management framework. KSII Trans. Internet Inf. Syst. **14**(3) (2020)

Guidelines to Develop an Art Therapy APP to Control the Children's State Anxiety in Mexico

Julieta Martínez, Marcela E. Buitrón(✉), and Edwing A. Almeida

Universidad Autónoma Metropolitana, Av. San Pablo 420, 02128 CDMX, México
{al2201800028,meb,eaac}@azc.uam.mx

Abstract. Anxiety state is a transitory condition that afflicts the child population of school age in Mexico City, whose control implies considering therapeutic treatments such as Art Therapy, a psycho therapeutic process that, through different artistic manifestations, offers available alternatives to control this disease. Although art therapies are usually carried out through analogous media and resources, the advances in mobile technology -as part of the implementation of the Internet of Things- and its easy children appropriation, have promoted the use of software applications as APP for mobile devices to optimize the therapeutic process. This requires identifying the contributions and opportunity areas of existing APPs for the Art Therapy process and propose approaches to define the guidelines to develop efficient applications for Art Therapy. This paper presents the justification and development process, based on a documental search and analysis of existing APPs, to propose guidelines to establish the conditions required for the development of an Art Therapy APP to support the therapeutic process in question.

Keywords: Child state anxiety · Art therapy · APP · IoT

1 Introduction

Anxiety state[1] is a transitory condition that is increasingly frequent in the school-age child population in Mexico City[2], which has a negative impact on the quality of life of those who suffer from it. To control this condition, there are various therapeutic[3] alternatives, among which Art Therapy stands out, as a form of psychotherapy that, according to the American Art Therapy Association (AATA), "uses active art-making, the creative process, and applied psychological theory —within a psychotherapeutic

---

[1] Spielberger (Schmidt and Shoji Muñoz 2018) defines state anxiety as a "transitory emotional condition of the human organism, which is characterized by subjective, consciously perceived feelings of tension and, as well as hyperactivity of the autonomic nervous system".

[2] According to the statistics of the National Institute of Statistics and Geography (INEGI 2017), the school-age child in Mexico City ranges from 6 to 11 years.

[3] Cognitive-behavioral therapies.

relationship— to enrich the lives of individuals" (American Art Therapy Association, 2022) from the contribution of certain benefits to the mental and emotional health of the patient. (Fig. 1).

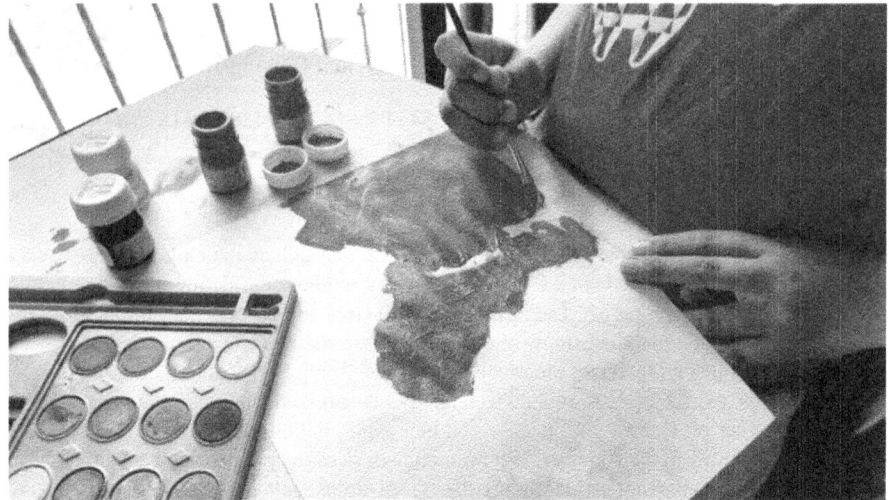

Fig. 1. Child Art Therapy

On a regular basis, art psychotherapies are carried out based on the development of therapeutic actions that involve certain artistic manifestations using different analogous media. However, advances in mobile technologies, advances in mobile technology, as part of the implementation of the Internet of things paradigm, and their rapid appropriation by infants, are promoting the use of software applications for mobile devices (APP) as resources to optimize the therapeutic process and, with this, offer alternatives to their development.

As a result, is possible to identify the existence of some medical APPs focused, through guided meditations, as well as the recording and monitoring of crises[4], to control anxiety in adults. However, in Mexico the existence of APPs that, since the development of actions typical of art therapy, support the therapeutic control of state anxiety, mainly focused on suffering in children, has not been documented yet[5].

This situation made latent the need to establish approaches that would identify the contributions of APPs to art therapy and, with this, be able to propose guidelines that, from actions related to the therapeutic act and the design of the digital resource, support its development.

---

[4] Martínez and Buitrón (2021) list, within this type of applications, Meyo©, IntelliCare Agora©, Drifting Afternoon©, Silk and Thisissand©, to mention a few.

[5] It should be noted that there aren´t scientific documents that support the use of art therapy APP to control the children's state anxiety in Mexico.

2 Methods

To develop a theoretical proposal that could respond to the mentioned problem,
should have been used a series of "methods and techniques for searching, processing and storing the information contained in [...] documents, [...] as well as the systematic, coherent presentation and sufficiently argued new information in a scientific document [...]" (Rizo 2015). The following Table 1 gives a summary of the actions followed for this purpose:

Table 1. Actions of documentary research.

Actions
Planning
Collection the information
Analysis and interpretation of the information
Results writing and presentation

Note: Actions defined from the methodological approach "Phases and techniques of documentary research", proposed by Janett Rizo Maradiaga (Rizo 2015)

3 Results

Based on the collection, analysis, and interpretation of a different authors[6] -experts in the topic- information, a series of guidelines have been proposed that establish the conditions required to develop an Art Therapy APP to support the therapeutic process in question.

3.1 Proposal Presentation

The control of children´s state of anxiety, being a transitory situation, can be achieved through cognitive-behavioral therapies, such as Arterial Therapy, which, based on different artistic manifestations and resources, allows carrying out actions for this purpose.

---

[6] Due to the lack of documented scientific work on the development of children's art therapy APP in Mexico, this proposal of guidelines, in congruence with the methods and techniques for their development, is based on the theoretical contributions of experts in Art Therapy and mobile application Design, such as: N. Choe (Choe 2014), C. Malchiodi (Malchiodi 2018) and E. Ronzón (Ronzón 2022) —design of APPs for children's mental health and art therapy—, in addition to J. Nielsen (Nielsen 2012), E. Mercovich (Mercovich 1999) and F. J. Fernández, (Fernández 2021) —usability and interfaces design—, and finally, companies and educational institutions such as PixSolution (PixSolution Hompage 2023), Yeeplay (Yeeply Hompage 2023) and ESDESIGN (ESDESIGN. Escuela superior de diseño de Barcelona Homepage 2023) — APP design—, which allowed to establish a series of approaches for the conformation of such design proposal.

In this sense and given the conditions that define children development in the current societies, the impact that the use of an APP -mobile technology derived from the implementation of the Internet of things paradigm, can have, as a digital therapeutic art resource, for the control of the disease, becomes evident.

This implies developing mobile applications considering certain guidelines related to the establishment of therapeutic conditions for the treatment in question, as well as the design of the APP and its ability to achieve therapeutic objectives (Fig. 2).

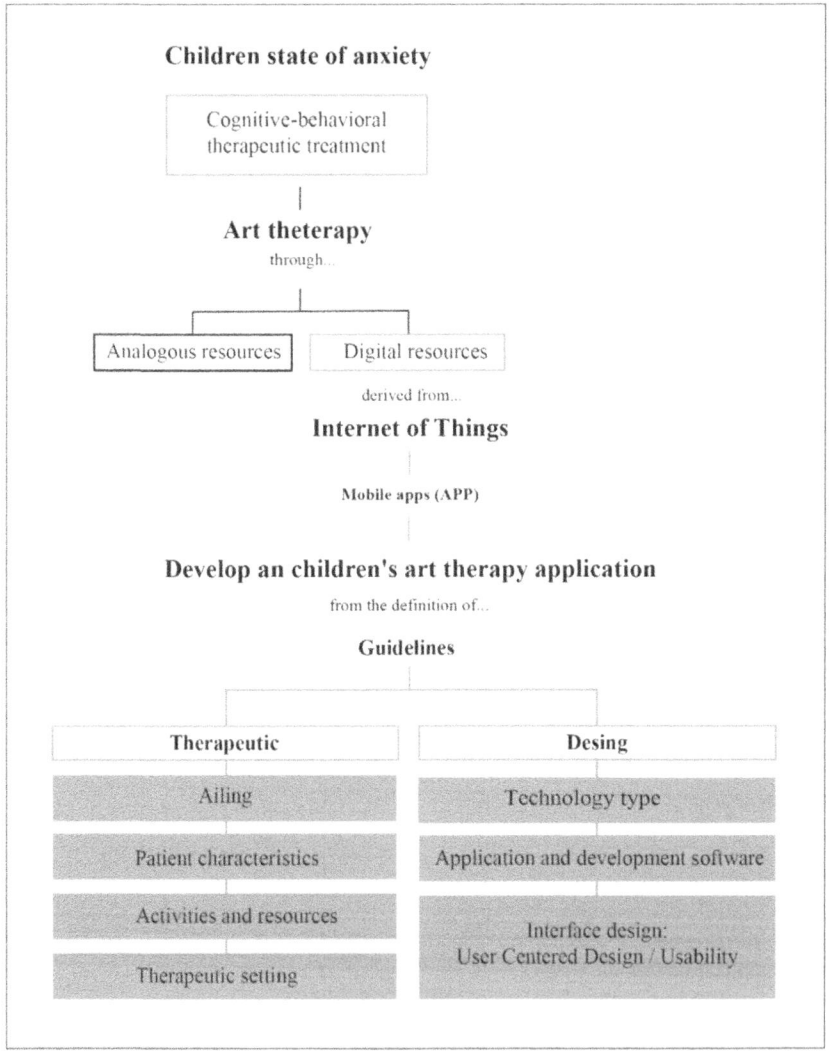

Fig. 2. Guidelines to develop a child's Art Therapy APP.

The development of an APP for children's art therapy must considerer those aspects that can identify the characteristics of the patient and the condition and based on this, define the necessary activities and resources, under a specific therapeutic framework. The therapeutic guidelines to consider are:

1. Recognize the condition, based on the therapist's diagnosis.
2. Identify the characteristics of the patient, in terms of age, sex, educational and socioeconomic level, among others.
3. Define the activities and therapeutic resources, depending on the condition and the characteristics of the type of patient.
4. Establish a therapeutic framework, reference to time, frequency, and rules of participation in therapeutic activities.

Also, they must require considerer aspects of the mobile application design, strengthening the ability to be efficiently used, such as:

1. Establish the technological feasibility, based on the technology choice to be the best suits in the therapeutic process.
2. Choose the operating system, according to technological feasibility, which will support the implementation of the APP, as well as its development.
3. Design the interface of the APP, considering those requirements for the activities and resources visualization, based on a design model focused on the characteristics and needs of its user, which may acquire the following capacities in its implementation: be useful for compliance with therapeutic fines; be easy to use, based on a clear understanding and retention of the parameters related to its operation; and, finally, to be able to generate perceptions, opinions, feelings and attitudes in the patient according to the therapeutic purposes.

It is considered that from the proposal of these guidelines it will be possible to define the necessary conditions to develop art therapy APPs that contribute significantly to the control of state anxiety in infants.

4 Conclusions

Given the increase in cases of state anxiety in children in Mexico, the application of art psychotherapy through technological resources, derived from the conditions that the presence of the Internet of Things imposes on the development of current societies, represents a good alternative for efficient therapeutic control of the disease.

The foregoing leads to be clear about the approaches that define the development of these mobile technologies, being able to conclude with the indication of the importance of considering guidelines related to both the therapeutic process, as well as the development of the APP itself, considering an action of design centered on the child patient, in such a way that this process is carried out efficiently in terms of achieving the expected therapeutic results.

Finally, although the efficiency of the proposed guidelines presented here can be validated based on the theoretical approaches put forward by various experts on the subject, the lack of documented case studies in Mexico may be a limitation to this effect.

This situation leads to the necessary consideration of a series of experimental processes to evaluate the effectiveness of each of the plans presented here, considering limitations ranging from a possible reconsideration of the choice of APPs as a means of disease control to an inadequate implementation of each of the guidelines proposed in their development.

References

American Art Therapy Association: About Art Therapy (2022). https:// arttherapy.org/about-art-therapy/. Accessed 13 May 2023

Choe, N.: An exploration of the qualities and features of art apps for art therapy. The Arts in Psychotherapy. **41**(2), 145–154 (2014). https://www.sciencedirect.com/science/article/abs/pii/S0197455614000033. 20 June 2020

ESDESIGN. Escuela superior de diseño de Barcelona Homepage, https://www.esdesignbarcelona.com/actualidad/diseno-web/todos-los-pasos-que-debes-seguir-para-crear-una-app-desde-cero. Acceded 16 Aug 2023

Fernández, J.F.: Utilización de Dispositivos Móviles Como Herramienta de Sensado en Aplicaciones de IoT (2021). http://sedici.unlp.edu.ar/handle/10915/121975. 13 May 2023

INEGI. Estadísticas a propósito del Día del niño (30 de abril) (2017). https://www.inegi.org.mx/contenidos/saladeprensa/aproposito/2017/nino2017_CdMx.docx. 10 July 2020

Malchiodi, C.A.: The handbook of Art Therapy and Digital Technology. Jessica Kingsley Publishers, Philadelphia (2018)

Martínez, J., Buitrón, M.E.: Visualización creativa de arteterapia a través de dispositivos digitales para reducir los niveles de ansiedad en preadolescentes en México. Investigación y Desarrollo - Reporte Fresnillo 2021, pp. 475–479 (2021). https://www.academiajournals.com/pubfresnillo2021. 23 Feb 2021

Mercovich, E.:. Diseño de Interfaces y Usabilidad: cómo hacer productos más útiles, eficientes y seductores. SIGGRAPH '99. Buenos Aires, Argentina (1999). 4http://planeta.gaiasur.com.ar/infoteca/siggraph99/diseno-de-interfaces-y-usabilidad.html. 10 Feb 2004

Nielsen, J.: Usability 101: Introduction to Usability, Nielsen Norman Group (2012). https://www.nngroup.com/articles/usability-101-introduction-to-usability/. 20 June 2020

PixSolution Homepage. https://www.pixsolution.tech/que-hace-que-una-aplicacion-sea-exitosa. Acceded 16 Aug 2023

Rizo, J.: Técnicas de Investigación Documental (2015). https://repositorio.unan.edu.ni/12168/1/100795.pdf. 20 June 2020

Ronzón, E.: Eliane Ronzón interview about Art Teraphy, by Julieta Martínez (2022). 25 Oct 2021

Yeeplay Hompage. https://www.yeeply.com/blog/diseno-de-aplicaciones-usabilidad-y-experiencia-de-usuario. Acceded 16 Aug 2023

Schmidt, V.P., Shoji Muñoz, A.D.: La ansiedad estado-rasgo y el rendimiento académico en adolescentes de 14 a 16 años. Degree Thesis in Educational Psychology, Universidad Católica Argentina, Facultad "Teresa de Ávila", Paraná (2018). http://bibliotecadigital.uca.edu.ar/greenstone/cgi-bin/library.cgi?a=d&c=tesis&d=ansiedad-estado-rasgo-rendimiento. 13 May 2023

Wearables in Healthcare

Commercial and Research-Based Wearable Devices in Spinal Postural Analysis: A Systematic Review

Narges Pourshahrokhi[(✉)], Yitong Sun, and Ali Asadipour

Computer Science Research Centre, Royal College of Art, London, UK
{narges.pourshahrokhi,ali.asadipour}@rca.ac.uk,
yitong.sun@network.rca.ac.uk

Abstract. The widespread use of ubiquitous computing has led to people spending more time in front of screens, causing poor posture. The COVID-19 pandemic and the shift towards remote work have only worsened the situation, as many people are now working from home with inadequate ergonomics. Maintaining a healthy posture is crucial for both physical and mental health, and poor posture can result in spinal problems. Wearable systems have been developed to monitor posture and provide instant feedback. Their goal is to improve posture over time by using these devices. This article will review commercially available, and research-based wearable devices used to analyse posture. The potential of these devices in the healthcare industry, particularly in preventing, monitoring, and treating spinal and musculoskeletal conditions, will also be discussed. The findings indicate that current devices can accurately assess posture in clinical settings, but further research is needed to validate the long-term effectiveness of these technologies and to improve their practicality for commercial use.

Keywords: Postural analysis · Wearable technology · Commercial devices · Spinal posture

1 Introduction

Having poor posture can affect both physical and mental health. Poor posture can lead to physical discomforts, such as back pain, neck pain, and shoulder pain, which can affect productivity. It can also lead to poor circulation and decreased oxygen intake, leading to fatigue and difficulty concentrating. Mentally, poor posture can affect self-esteem and confidence. Standing or sitting with poor posture can give off the appearance of being unconfident or disinterested, which can negatively impact social interactions and opportunities. Poor posture can also lead to poor sleep quality, as it can cause discomfort and difficulty finding a comfortable position. In addition, poor posture can lead to long-term health problems, such as arthritis, osteoporosis, and degenerative joint diseases, which can significantly impact the overall quality of life. Therefore, poor posture can have significant negative impacts on both physical and mental health, and it is important to strive for good posture in order to avoid these disadvantages [16, 33, 51, 52].

Moreover, the term "posture" is often used in the context of sports and fitness, and health but the definition of this term can be quite vague and subjective. There are a variety of different factors that can contribute to poor spine posture, including muscle imbalances, poor core stability, and improper technique. This lack of clarity makes it difficult for coaches, athletes, medical experts, and researchers to accurately identify and correct poor spine posture, which can negatively impact performance and overall health.

One of the main challenges with defining poor spine posture is that it can vary depending on an individual's body type and physical abilities. Some individuals may have naturally fine spine posture due to their physical structure and muscle balance, while others may struggle with poor spine posture due to previous injuries or other physical limitations. This means that what constitutes poor spine posture for one person may not necessarily be the same for another, making it difficult to establish a clear and consistent definition.

Another issue with the definition of posture is that it can be influenced by a variety of different factors. For instance, poor spine posture can caused by muscle imbalances, where certain muscles are overdeveloped while others are underdeveloped. This can lead to poor alignment and stability, which can make it difficult to maintain good spine posture. Additionally, poor core stability can also contribute to poor spine posture, as the core muscles play a crucial role in maintaining proper alignment and balance.

The definition of posture can vary depending on the specific activity in which it is being applied. For example, in sports such as tennis, a good spine posture might involve a wide stance and a bent knee in order to generate power and control on shots. In contrast, the office working environment posture can be defined as the angle that hands make while resting on the table or the angle of the neck while looking at the screen.

It is crucial to identify poor posture early and maintain good posture to prevent injuries and the development of spinal disease. In medical field, human posture is assessed by the Bath Ankylosing Spondylitis Metrology Index (BASMI) using a measuring tape and goniometers to obtain the measurements. Incorrect use of the instruments, erratic or compensatory movements of the subject or observation errors can appear, which can cause a lack of accuracy and reproducibility [11, 43, 45]. On the other hand, the spine and sacroiliac joints create complicated motions that cannot be analysed using the BASMI approach. As a result, it is critical to research and develop new technology-based posture estimation techniques that can assess joints directly with acceptable accuracy, repeatability, and sensitivity to changes in information over time.

The human spine consists of 33 individual vertebrae separated by intervertebral discs and grouped into five regions: the cervical, thoracic, lumbar, sacral, and coccygeal regions. Each vertebra has a unique shape and size, with the cervical region having smaller and more mobile vertebrae than the lumbar region.

As shown in Fig. 1, the cervical spine is the portion of the spine within the neck, and consists of 7 vertebrae (C1 to C7).

The 12 thoracic vertebrae (T1 to T12) are contained within the rib cage, and each vertebra articulates with a rib. These are far less mobile, and this more rigid structure of the thoracic spine provides the necessary support for the vital organs contained in the chest (heart and lungs). The lumbar spine is the lowest mobile segment and is commonly referred to as the lower back. It has 5 vertebrae (L1 to L5), and these are the largest vertebrae in the spine as they have the greatest load to bear.

Optical marker-based devices are a widely used technology for tracking motion and evaluating spinal mobility, but they have certain limitations in clinical settings due to their high cost, indoor-only capabilities, and need for specific equipment and conditions [4,6,21]. Researchers have attempted to overcome these issues by using technologies such as inertial measurement unit (IMU) to create wearable capture devices for human posture modelling [17,20,36,75]. These wearables are more cost-effective and can be used in any location without the need for a complex setup.

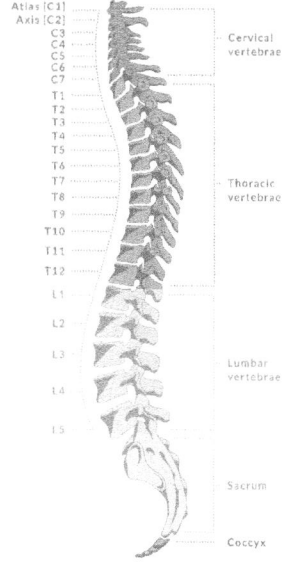

Fig. 1. Human Spine labelled with the joins name and group

Wearables are also widespread in the industrial and commercial markets for assisting users in improving their quality of life. For instance, they provide continuous and personalised health monitoring, physical activity, and vital signs while offering features like stress tracking, GPS tracking, and hands-free access to notifications and calls. Wearable devices for tracking spinal disorders during daily activity as an indication of health status are a trending venue for healthcare. With 239 million units in demand worldwide and over 1.2 billion devices expected to be in use by the end of 2025, with yearly sales approaching 400 million units in the year, the market forecast for wearables is optimistic [3,59]. Therefore employing wearables for spinedisorder and correction feedback appears promising from a business perspective.

The introduction of new wearables and new sensor technologies has dramatically exceeded the limitations of traditional data capture methods, making it possible to acquire significant amounts of data [57]. However, with emergence of more complex data and gradual sharing of various clinical data sets, the sample size and potential predictor variables can exceed tens of thousands [44]. Traditional data analysis methods can no longer cope effectively, so alternative methods (e.g. complex data analysis) are needed to process such large amounts of information. Moreover, the fact that humans often present a much more complex posture in everyday life than in experimental settings has led to the validity of some of the datasets being questioned in practical applications [49]. As a result, one of the most critical challenges today is consistently collecting valid data over extended periods in complex environments outside the laboratory.

Machine learning (ML) has been shown to outperform classical computational methods in various tasks, including big data processing, data prediction, posture perdiction and object detection, thanks to rapid development of Artificial Intelligence (AI) field [5,30]. A subset of ML, Deep Learning (DL), has led to significant advances and accuracy improvements in 2D human posture estimation tasks based on images and single-frame sequences [46]. The use of ML-derived algorithms and data models can enable the faster conversion of diverse and large databases into low resource-consuming applications on low-cost devices (e.g., smartphones, tablets, laptops) [34,62], save significant manual time, and circumvent potential errors caused by humans to aid faster and more accurate real-time decision-making.

Furthermore, some studies have used multi-stage classification models to improve the recognition of complex postures. These models have achieved satisfactory accuracy rates in specific pose acquisition and localised body recognition. However, there are still significant limitations in full-body generic pose acquisition and in collecting data in complex environments in the real life. Several studies on postural assessment have also been developed. Wu et al. [77] proposed three criteria, namely joint angle, arm orientation and type of joint motion, that could be used to assess the forearm and upper arm. Khachai et al. [25] proposed a postural description language to redefine human posture and assess whole-body motion. However, they are difficult to assess quantitatively for non-standard body parts and have not been applied to a generalised postural assessment of the whole body. Meanwhile, ethicists have also raised risks and concerns about using ML for individual assessment and decision-making [15,39,65]. The risks are not only limited to a widespread lack of transparency in the data sets used for modelling, but the credibility of the decisions made cannot be validated as there is no uniform standard for posture assessment. The purpose of this systematic review is to carefully review and compare the recent advances and shortcomings in the use of wearable devices for estimating spinal posture, and to identify areas for further research and development. The specific research questions considered are as follows:

- **RQ1.** What are the recent studies and commercial wearable devices for Musculoskeletal posture detection?
- **RQ2.** Are these wearable devices practical in a real-world setting?
- **RQ3.** What are the limitations of the devices that capture human Musculoskeletal posture?

- **RQ4.** What are the data analysis methods used for estimating Musculoskeletal posture?
 - **RQ5.** How can ML techniques contribute to estimating and assessing human Musculoskeletal posture?

2 Method

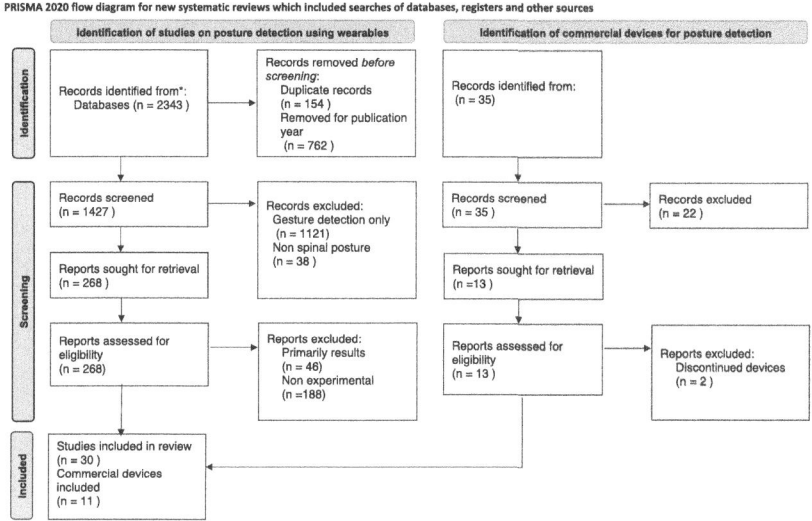

Fig. 2. PRISMA flowchart on academic and commercial wearable devices to estimate spinal posture

For this systematic review, the Reporting Items for Systematic Reviews and Meta Analyses Guidelines (PRISMA) were employed across five sources, namely: PubMed, MEDLINE, EMBASE, Cochrane, and Scopus. Following a general screening with a list of suitable key phrases, the final selection of key search terms was taken from pre-established headings on the OVID Medline (Med-line) database. Among the key search phrases were: ("human spine posture") AND ("recognition" OR "estimation" OR "evaluation" OR "capture") AND ("artificial Intelligence" OR "machine learning" OR "deep learning") AND ("wearable" , "sensor"). Spelling variants and synonyms were included and updated for each database as needed. Figure 2 depicts the PRISMA flow chart. The search results were limited to studies that met the following inclusion criteria:

Table 1. Summary of outcome from reviewed articlessss

Reference	Sensor	Region of Interest	Feedback System	# of participants	Environment	Data Analysis Method	Evaluation/validation	Posture definition
Bartalesi, R et al. 2010 [7]	Textile based piezoresistive sensor, IMU (3 DOF)	1: sacrum 2: spinous 3: T 12	No real-time feedback	–	Laboratory	measuring the correlation coefficient with the reference signal	Estimate error with reference signal	The curvature of lower back
O'Sullivan K, et al. 2012 [55]	BodyGuard: strain gauge	L3 to S2	Real-time biofeedback	12	Laboratory	Correlation in measurements	Comparing with marker-based motion analysis (video fluoroscopy)	Percentage of strain gauge elongation relative to range of motion (ROM), Pilot Study
Gopalai A, et al. 2012 [24]	MicroStrain's wireless IMU	1: Attached to trunk via waist band, 2: wobble board.	Real-time vibrotactile feedback	10	Laboratory	fuzzy logic based artificial intelligent system		Euler angular measurements trunk angle and wobble board angle Pilot study inspired by [26]
Lou E, et al. 2012 [40]	Smart garment	1: upper back 2: lower back.	Real-time vibrotactile feedback	1	Laboratory	correlation and difference between measured angles form proposed device and validation methods	Comparing with rotating wheel in static set up, and optical motion device in dynamic setup	Measurement of the kyphotic angle [41]
Wu W, et al. 2014 [76]	IMU (3 DOF)	Vest containing: 1: below neck, 2: chest, 3: centre of mass, 4: left hip, 5: right hip	No real-time feedback	10	Laboratory	Linear transfomation	Angle error computed by proposed method	Tilt angles from single IMU (3 DOF) on vest [38]
Tsuchiya Y, et al. 2014 [67]	Flex sensor, IMU (3 DOF)	Upper lumbar spine and sacrum, flex sensors between.	No real-time feedback	20	Laboratory	The cumulative error value of body coordinates	Compared to corresponding body coordinates from X-ray image	The center of gravity in the upper body and the waist shape [69]
Sardini E, et al. 2015 [63]	Inductive sensor	Inductive sensor sewn to the back and front shirt.	Real-time vibrotactile feedback	24	Laboratory	correlation coefficient and mean difference	Comparing with the optical system	Runk in the sagittal plane, and percentage of the Range of Motion (ROM) [29,54]
Miyajima S, et al. 2015 [48]	IMU (6 DOF)	1: lumbar spine 2: thigh 3: calf	No real-time feedback	4	Laboratory/ Home	angle error in estimation of joint angle	Compared to SIMM[thre ref]	Estimating joint torque using three link angles of the body, thigh, and shank [2]
Gleadhill S, et al. 2016 [23]	SABEL Sense IMU (3 DOF)	1: C7, 2: T1, 2, 3: S1	No real-time feedback	11	Laboratory	Will Hopkins Typical Error, Pearson correlation, Bland Altman Limits of agreement	Comparing with 3D MoCap	–
Ribeiro D, et al.2016 [60]	Spineangel (IMU 6 DOF)	Attached to belt .	Real-time auditory alarm	4	In the Field	covariate measurement controlling with baseline inubalance	Evaluation with the Oswestry Disability Index (ODI)	Threshold of cumulative forward flexed trunk posture [61]
Lin W, et al.2016 [37]	IMU (3 DOF)	1: lower cervical spine 2: middle of the chest 3: L3 (centre of mass) 4: right waist 5: left waist.	Real-time feedback via smartphone	–	–	maxumum error measured.	The maximum error of the tilting angle transformation using validation test [19]	The tilting angles of critical locations of the body [38]
Voinea G, et al.2016 [71]	IMU (9 DOF)	Sensors affixed to shirt in upper thoracic to lower lumbar spine	No real-time feedback	40	Laboratory	cumulative error	Error from the mathematical model was measured in C2 and A4 posture in reconstruction	Measuring orientation angles to represents the curvature of the spine
Nath N, et al. 2017 [53]	Smartphone IMU (6 DOF)	1: upper arm 2: waist	No real-time feedback	16	Simulated working environment	an equation to measure trunk and shoulder flexions based on angular features	Comparing with observation-based measurements. Metric: minimum absolute errors	Angular rotations of different body parts [42]
Fathi A, et al. 2017 [19]	Shimmer IMU (6 DOF)	1: cervical spine 2: thoracic spine 3: lower lumbar spine.	Real-time feedback	–	Laboratory	Symbolic Aggregate approXimation	Metric: minimum lower bounding distance, and classification accuracy	Ankylosing spondylitis Hunchback and slouching back [1]
Valdivia S, et al. 2017 [70]	IMU (9 DOF)	waist	Real-time feedback via exergame	5	Laboratory	focused on System Usability Scale score rather than posture itself	Comparing with kintect version2 in terms of flexion angle measurement	Flexion angle [22]
Xu J, et al. 2017 [78]	IMU (9 DOF) InvenSense	Eight IMUs placed on left and right sides of torso at L4/L5	Real-time vibrotactile feedback	–	Laboratory	statistical significants	RMS and percentage of time inside no zone while using system vs not using system	Used balance posture term by measuring trunk tilt and foot rotation angle [31].
Hansraj K, et al. 2017 [27]	SPoMo (IMU 6 DOF)	1: upper back 2: lower back.	Real-time vibrotactile feedback	4	Laboratory	measuring Force To Cervical Spine at specific neck angles	Using Cosmosworks software, a finite element assessment package	The ears alignment with the shoulders and the angel wings or the shoulder blades [13, 28, 72]
Cornea, G et al. 2018 [61]	IMU (9 DOF)	5 sensors along spine	No real-time feedback	–	Laboratory	Mathematical model based on circle arcs	calculating the radius and the coordinates of the IMU sensors	circle arcs and radius model of spine to match its X-ray
Lim C, et al. 2018 [35]	IMU (3 DOF)	1: Lumber 2: cervical spine.	No real-time feedback	3	Laboratory	Error estimation in measuring angles	Comparing with goniometer and electrogoniometer	Calculation of the angle
Wang, Z, et al. 2019 [73]	IMU (9 DOF)	3 sensors on lower lumbar spine	No Real-time feedback	15	Laboratory, Swimming pool	An algorithm to combine orientation estimation with the human biomechanical model	Comparing with the NDI motion tracking system	Equilateral triangle bracket structure in the horizontal plane
Bootsman, R et al. 2019 [10]	Smart garmentIMU (9 DOF) Lumo Back	Lower spine	Real-time feedback	60	Hospital	Qualitative data analysis	Three validated questionnaires	Lumbar flexion measurement

(continued)

Table 1. (*continued*)

Reference	Sensor	Region of Interest	Feedback System	# of participants	Environment	Data Analysis Method	Evaluation/validation	Posture definition
Stollenwerk, K et al. 2019 [66]	SpineTracker	Between C7 and L4 vertebrae	Real-time feedback	360	Laboratory	The cumulative error value of body coordinates	Compared to corresponding body coordinates from X-ray image	The center of gravity in the upper body and the waist shape [69]
Cavicdes, J, et al. 2020 [14]	StretchSense: strain gauge	upside-down triangle of sensors on posterior torso	Real-time biofeedback	6	Laboratory	a single class classifier	Sum of the Point-wise Mahalanobis Distances (SPMD)	curvature of spine inspired by specialised PT exercise therapy, Pilot Study
Wielgos, S et al. 2020 [74]	Magnetic sensors	On grid shirt align with spine	No Real-time feedback	4	Laboratory	Simulated curvatures of the spine	Preliminary results based on angle measurement	Measuring angles
Conforti, I et al. 2020 [18]	IMU (6 DOF)	Suprasternal notch, Pelvis, mid-thighs, mid-shanks, instep of the feet	No real-time feedback	26	Laboratory, Working Environment	Support vector machine	Accuracy in classification	range of motion of lower limb lumbosacral joint displacement of the trunk
Petropoulos, A et al. 2020 [58]	IMU (6 DOF)	1: upper back 2: lowerback	No real-time feedback	-	Laboratory	Angle error in estimation	Reporting RMSE in angle estimation	Estimating angle between lower and upper sensor parallel with spine
Kuo, Y et al. 2021 [32]	Lumo Lift	belowclavicle, and midway between the sternal notch	Real-time feedback	21	Laboratory	Correlation in measurement	Comparing with Vicon Motion system	Joint angles segment inclination angles, and pelvic plane angles
Carbonaro, N et al. 2021 [12]	IMU (9 DOF)	sacral level thoracic levelhead level	Real-time vibrotactile feedback	1	Operatory room	Qualitative data analysis	RULA scoring	flexion, lateral bending, and twisting angles of spine and neck
Michaud F, et al. 2022 [47]	IMU (9 DOF)	T1, T4, T7, T10L1, L5	No real-time feedback	14	Laboratory	Measuring location of sensors and estimated position of sensor	Comparing with optical motion capture	3D human spine estimation through a subject-specific multibody model
Moon, K, et al. 2023 [50]	IMU (6 DOF)	pelvis, Two on either is of spine	No real-time feedback	1	Laboratory	Error estimation in measuring angles	Estimation of the matching error level from the predetermined template motion obtained from the robotic simulator	Calculation of 3D angles of the hip and spine in the sagittal

– Articles involving wearable technologies which are able to monitor posture of human
– Data analysis methods were used for data analysis
– Control group experiments or accuracy validation were available
– Article published after 2010
– Articles written in English

We also have excluded following criteria from our screening:

– Articles that are only capable of identifying body positions such as walking, sitting, lying down
– Wearable technology that focus on monitoring posture parts other than spine

The initial database search yielded 2343 potentially relevant articles; however, 154 duplicates were excluded. After applying inclusion and exclusion criteria, 1159 articles were eliminated. The remaining 268 titles and abstracts were then scanned to identify potentially relevant studies. Of these, 234 did not meet the inclusion criteria due to: preliminary results (n=46), and non-experimental studies (n=188). As a result, data were extracted from 30 studies that met the inclusion and exclusion criteria.

After scanning chosen publications for bias using the Newcastle-Ottawa Scale of Quality Assessment. We explored the selected articles in terms of sensor technology, region of interest, feedback presents, participant number, lab or real-world setting, data analysis technique, assessment method, and the posture definition employed. Table 1 provides a thorough summary of the outcome.

Furthermore, another inquiry on Google and Espacenet was conducted to uncover the commercially available posture wearable technology. This study

Table 2. Commercial Devices for Spinal Posture detection

	Upright Go S	Upright Go 2	LumoBack	Alex	Nadi X	Sense-U	ZiktoWalk	Prana	Jins Meme	Sensoria	postureTracker
Size (mm)	48 × 28	48 × 28	415 × 100	80 × 160	NA	35.6 × 35.6	13.6 × 47.3	31.8 × 6.4	NA	33 x 33	33 × 16
Weight (g)	12	11	25	25	NA	11.34	17.5	NA	36	7	10
Sensor location	Upper Back	Upper Back	Waist	Neck	Hips, knees, ankles	Clavicle	Waist	Waist	Nose bridge, ears	Foot, Upper Back	Lower back
Battery life (hours)	12	20	120	168	1.5	240	120	168	16	20	20
Feedback System	Visuo-haptic	Visuo-haptic	Visuo-haptic	Visual	Visuo-haptic	Visual	Visual	Visual	Visual	No Feedback	Visual
Data availability	No	No	No	No	No	No	No	No	No	Yes	Yes

found and used 11 commercially available posture devices in total. "posture", "wearable", "device", and "commercial" were utilised as search phrases. Wearables with posture-recording and monitoring capabilities met the inclusion requirements; however, devices that mechanically adjusted posture, like braces, or products whose device specs were unknown or unavailable were among the exclusion criteria. As demonstrated in Fig. 2, the results of this investigation were contributed to the PRISMA as additional source of search results.

3 Findings

The study conducted a comprehensive review of 30 articles selected from a total of 2343 papers on human posture analysis. Out of the 30 selected articles, 14 (46%) used distance error measurement, 8 (26%) used model approximation, 5 (16%) used artificial intelligence, 2 (6%) used usability metric, and only 1 (3%) used qualitative measurements for their data analysis.

In terms of the experimental setting, most experiments were conducted in a laboratory environment (74%), 7 (23%) were conducted in a working environment, and the remaining experiment (3%) did not specify the environment setting. The acquisition points for human posture analysis varied from one local point to 20 points, with the majority of studies (83%) focusing on the spinal area for sensor placement. Additionally, 2 studies (6%) used a modified shirt, the same number of studies used an upside-down triangle shape for sensor placement, and one study (3%) used a belt for sensor placement.

In terms of sensor technology, the majority of studies (70%) used IMU sensors, 5 (16%) used commercial devices, 2 (6%) used strain gauge, 1 used textile, and 1 used a smart garment. The number of participants in the experiments varied from 1 to 360, with some studies not specifying the case study size. The definition of posture was not uniform, with each study defining it differently.

The study also reviewed 11 commercial devices, investigating their size, weight, body placement, presence of a feedback system, availability of collected data for researchers, and the presence of research studies. In terms of weight, wearables ranged from 7g to 36g. only 2 (18%) didn't specify the weight of the device. In terms of sensor placement, 3 (27%) focused on the upper body, 3 (27%) targeted the waist, and the rest aimed at the Neck, Clavicle, Nose ridge, ear, lower back, and foot. The battery life of the wearables covered a range of 1.5 h to 168 h. Regarding the presence of a feedback system, most devices (90%) had Mobile application feedback. In terms of the availability of data for researchers, only 2 (18%) had data available for other researchers to use. The details and features of commercial devices are available in Table 2.

4 Discussion

Wearables that monitor posture have the ability to prevent developing poor posture by providing real-time feedback and promoting the correction of poor posture. Many prototypes capable of assessing spinal position have been presented in the literature. A diverse set of technologies supports these systems. IMUs are the most regularly utilised, offering 3 to 10 Degrees of Freedom (DOF). Strain gauges, flex sensors, fibre-optic goniometers, inductive sensors, and ergonomic dosimeters are some other technologies employed in posture monitoring wearables [8,9,56,64,68]. A comparative detail of the studies is presented in Tables 1 and 2. This section discusses the details and our findings from the reviewed resources.

4.1 Posture Definition

The definition of posture that each research study selected was surprisingly broad. While two studies developed their own unique definitions of posture and tested them in pilot studies, the majority employed some form of angular measurement to assess posture. However, the specific location and the combinations of angles and set-ups varied across studies. Defining posture presents a challenge as it is contingent on the underlying causes of poor posture, thereby influencing how it is measured. It is essential for the literature to establish a clear and standardised definition of posture to facilitate measurement and enable researchers to utilise a unified metric for comparing different models. However, the current wide range of methodological approaches for measuring posture presents a challenge in this regard. Comparing studies that use various measures for defining posture is difficult, given the lack of a standardised definition.

4.2 Sensor Technology

An Inertial Measurement Unit (IMU) is a device that consists of sensors that measure acceleration, angular velocity, and sometimes magnetic field strength. These sensors can be used to determine the orientation, position, and movement of an object. IMUs are often used in wearable devices for posture detection because they are small, lightweight, and can operate without the need for external references. Several types of sensors are commonly used in IMUs, including accelerometers, gyroscopes, and magnetometers. Each of these sensors measures a different physical quantity, and the data from these sensors can be combined using algorithms to determine the orientation and movement of the device. The degrees of freedom (DOF) in IMU sensors refer to the number of independent axes along which an object's motion can be measured. Generally, an IMU sensor can have 3, 6, or 9 DOF. A 3 DOF IMU can measure acceleration along the three axes of X, Y, and Z, while a 6 DOF IMU can measure both acceleration and rotational velocity around these three axes. On the other hand, a 9 DOF IMU can measure all three axes of acceleration, rotational velocity, and the direction of the Earth's magnetic field. Generally, a higher number of DOF in an IMU sensor means more accurate measurements of an object's motion and orientation. Only 4 (13%) publications in this systematic review used IMU with 3 DOF, The majority, however, used IMU with 6 DOF that is possibly due to factors such as cost, power consumption, application requirements, and simplicity of data processing. 12 (40%) publications measured the posture concurrently with a combination of two to three sensors along with IMU. Three studies exclusively employed texture and pressure sensors, whereas one research incorporated an optical sensor (light).

4.3 Sensor Placement

Wearable placement of the body was an interesting aspect of this systematic review. While the majority of studies considered curvature and the spine's structure related to poor posture, each of them chose various spine locations for measurement.

14% of studies focused on the cervical, 21% targeted the sacrum and 28% aimed at Lumar, while the majority (35%) of studies considered the thoracal region of the spine for their measurement.

4.4 Environmental Setting

Experimental studies often rely on controlled environments to minimise confounding variables' influence and ensure that the results are reproducible. This is why many experiments are conducted indoors and in laboratory settings. In these controlled settings, researchers can carefully manipulate the independent variables and measure their effects on the dependent variables while keeping other variables constant. Additionally, laboratory equipment and instruments can be calibrated and standardised to reduce measurement errors, which is particularly important when conducting high-precision experiments. However, the controlled nature of laboratory experiments also limits their ecological validity or the extent to which the results can be generalised to real-life situations. Furthermore, laboratory equipment and facilities can be expensive or impractical for real-life usage. While laboratory experiments have their advantages, they may not always be practical or feasible when studying phenomena that occur in the real world or in outdoor environments. However, outdoor experiments also present many challenges, such as the lack of control over environmental conditions, difficulty in replicating the same conditions across multiple experiments, and the potential for confounding variables to influence the results. As a result, experimental designs for outdoor settings often involve compromises between control and ecological validity. In this systematic review majority, (84%) of experiments were conducted in a laboratory and controlled environment only five (16 %) experiments were adapted to real-life experience. It is necessary to design practical wearables in real work to be helpful and impactful.

4.5 Data Availability

In this systematic review, we observed that data for other researchers were only available in some cases. Publicly available data can encourage further analysis and replication of the findings. It also helps researchers in the field to improve existing work and develop more optimised outcomes. This can be particularly important in posture detection and public health, where access to data can inform policy decisions and lead to improvements in people's care. However, in other cases, the data may be restricted due to privacy concerns or ownership issues. However, the data may be restricted in other cases due to privacy concerns or ownership issues. For example, wearable technology such as fitness trackers or smartwatches can collect large amounts of data on individuals' health and behaviour, but this data may be subject to privacy laws or the terms of service of the device manufacturer. The lack of availability of data from wearable technology can pose challenges for researchers who are interested in studying health or behaviour. While wearable devices can provide valuable insights into individuals' activity, spine structure, and posture, access to this data may be limited by factors such as cost, privacy concerns, or proprietary algorithms. This can create barriers to replicating studies or conducting meta-analyses, which rely on the availability of large datasets. Additionally, the ownership of the data may be unclear, which can make it difficult for researchers to obtain permission to use the data or to share it with other researchers.

4.6 Data Analysis

In terms of data analysis, while existing and reviewed papers had valuable tools for evidence-based decision-making, the data analysis methods used in these reviews are often relatively basic. This can limit the accuracy of the outcome, as it may not fully capture the nuances of the underlying data. One potential way to improve the accuracy of systematic reviews is by incorporating AI and ML techniques. AI and ML can be used to analyse large datasets and identify patterns that may not be immediately apparent using traditional statistical methods. This can help to increase the accuracy of the outcome by providing a more nuanced understanding of the data. AI and ML can be particularly useful in scenarios with wearables that often involve significant and complex datasets. This can help to identify gaps or inconsistencies in the literature and provide insights into areas that may require further research.

5 Beneficiary in Well-Being and Healthcare

Wearable technologies have the potential to revolutionise the way we monitor and improve our health and well-being, and one area where they have made significant strides is in the detection of human posture. These technologies can be used to not only identify poor posture, but also provide feedback and coaching to help individuals improve their posture and reduce the risk of injury or pain. In this systematic review, we also explore the application of wearable technologies for human posture detection and the benefits they offer for both individuals and healthcare professionals.

One of the primary benefits of wearable technologies for human posture detection is their ability to continuously monitor posture throughout the day. Traditional methods of posture assessment, such as manual observation or static photographs, are limited in their ability to capture posture changes over time or in different positions. Wearable technologies, on the other hand, can track posture in real-time, allowing for a more comprehensive understanding of an individual's posture habits and patterns.

One of the most significant advantages of wearable devices is their potential to facilitate behavioural modification and promote positive lifestyle changes. By continuously monitoring posture habits, these devices create a feedback loop that encourages individuals to adopt healthier postural habits in their daily lives. As users become more conscious of their posture, they are likely to make conscious choices to prioritise good posture, not just during device usage but throughout their day-to-day activities. This behavioural modification can extend beyond posture, leading to increased awareness of overall health and well-being.

In addition to providing individuals with a convenient and accurate way to monitor their posture, wearable technologies for posture detection also offer benefits for healthcare professionals. By providing continuous posture data, these technologies can help healthcare professionals identify patterns and risk factors for injury or pain, and provide more targeted interventions and treatment plans. For example, a physical therapist working with a patient who suffers from chronic back pain could use wearable posture detection technology to identify specific postures or activities that may be contributing to the patient's pain, and develop a treatment plan based on this information. Moreover, using vision-based technology has raised concerns about the potential invasion of privacy, as they can capture personal information and activities without the individual's consent. Additionally, cameras can be hacked or accessed without the owner's knowledge, putting them at risk of cyber attacks or identity theft. Unlike vision-based technology, wearables do not capture visual data and instead rely on sensors to collect information. Thus, using wearables can maintain the benefits of technology while protecting privacy, making them a viable alternative to vision-based technology.

The boundary between smart health wearables and medical devices is becoming blurred with advancements in technology, allowing patients to take a more active role in their health and manage ongoing conditions. However, the use of commercial wearables in healthcare has both benefits and drawbacks. Healthcare professionals may be overwhelmed with the increase of patients bringing their own data to appointments, leading to confusion and tension. Alternatively, healthcare professionals and researchers could collaborate to validate wearable devices as a supportive tool in the healthcare system.

The use of wearable technology in the field of spine posture analysis offers several potential benefits, including:

- Early Detection of Postural Issues: Wearable technology enables real-time monitoring of spinal posture, which allows for early detection of postural issues. Early detection of these issues can lead to prompt intervention and prevent more serious problems from developing in the future.
- Improved Treatment Outcomes: By providing more accurate and detailed information about spinal posture, wearable technology can lead to improved treatment outcomes for individuals suffering from back pain, spinal injuries, or other postural problems.
- Increased Accessibility: Wearable technology offers an affordable and accessible solution for individuals to monitor their spinal posture, regardless of their location or access to healthcare facilities. This increased accessibility can lead to earlier and more effective treatment for postural issues.
- Better Understanding of Spinal Mechanics: Wearable technology can provide valuable data on spinal mechanics, which can help medical professionals better understand the causes of postural issues and develop more effective treatments.
- Improved Compliance: Wearable technology can provide real-time feedback on posture, which can encourage individuals to adopt better postural habits and improve compliance with treatment plans.

The use of wearables in healthcare is still in its early stages, and its potential applications and limitations are yet to be fully understood. Wearable technology has the potential to offer numerous benefits to healthcare providers and individuals alike. By enabling real-time monitoring and improved understanding of spinal mechanics, wearable technology can help prevent and treat postural problems, leading to improved health outcomes for individuals.

6 Conclusion

This paper has reviewed the current state of the art in wearable devices for monitoring and detecting spinal posture, as well as commercial devices. The current method for analysing posture is through radiography, but optical methods are emerging as a potential alternative. This paper shows that despite the benefits of using various technologies to measure posture, more research is needed to improve their accuracy, determine their clinical usefulness, and enhance their practicality before they can be widely adopted.

Furthermore, these laboratory-based methods are not suitable for daily posture monitoring. Wearable technology could fill this gap by providing objective measurements of posture. However, the lack of standardisation in posture definitions remains a challenge. Although there is a growing trend of commercial wearable devices using IMUs for continuous data collection, more research is needed to confirm their validity. Their data could potentially be used to detect spinal conditions earlier and more easily.

Our review highlights the advances made in this field, as well as the limitations that must be considered when designing and evaluating these devices. We have also identified several key concerns, including the availability of data, restrictions in experiment environment settings, data analysis, sensor technology and placement, and the potential application of these devices in healthcare.

One of the key challenges facing researchers and practitioners in this field is the need to balance the advantages of wearable devices with the limitations that arise from their use. While wearable devices offer many potential benefits, such as increased accuracy and real-time monitoring, they are also subject to limitations, such as the standardised definition of posture and employing AI for data analysis. Future research should continue to address these challenges and work towards developing more reliable and accurate wearable devices for monitoring spinal posture.

Overall, the findings of this paper emphasise the need for continued innovation in wearable technology, with a particular focus on the development of devices that can be used in various environmental settings, provide reliable and accurate data, and have clear applications in healthcare. By addressing these concerns, researchers and practitioners can work towards developing more effective interventions for spinal posture monitoring and detection, with the potential to improve patient outcomes and quality of life.

Acknowledgment. This research is funded by the Laboratory for Artificial Intelligence in Design (Project Code: RP1-6) under the InnoHK Research Clusters, Hong Kong Special Administrative Region Government.

References

1. Basdai bath ankylosing spondylitis disease activity index. https://www.basdai.com/
2. Va technical reference model v 22.11. https://www.oit.va.gov/Services/TRM
3. Adams, S.: Healthy outlook for wearables as users focus on fitness and well-being (2022). https://www.ccsinsight.com/company-news/healthy-outlook-for-wearables-as-users-focus-on-fitness-and-well-being/
4. Aghazadeh, F., Arjmand, N., Nasrabadi, A.: Coupled artificial neural networks to estimate 3d whole-body posture, lumbosacral moments, and spinal loads during load-handling activities. J. Biomech. **102**, 109332 (2020)
5. Alzubi, J., Nayyar, A., Kumar, A.: Machine learning from theory to algorithms: an overview. J. Phys.: Conf. Ser. **1142**, 012012 (2018). IOP Publishing
6. Asadi, F., Arjmand, N.: Marker-less versus marker-based driven musculoskeletal models of the spine during static load-handling activities. J. Biomech. **112**, 110043 (2020)
7. Bartalesi, R., Lorussi, F., De Rossi, D., Tesconi, M., Tognetti, A.: Wearable monitoring of lumbar spine curvature by inertial and e-textile sensory fusion. In: 2010 Annual International Conference of the IEEE Engineering in Medicine and Biology, pp. 6373–6376. IEEE (2010)

8. Bell, J., Stigant, M.: Development of a fibre optic goniometer system to measure lumbar and hip movement to detect activities and their lumbar postures. J. Med. Eng. Technol. **31**(5), 361–366 (2007)
9. Bhattacharya, A., Warren, J., Teuschler, J., Dimov, M., Medvedovic, M., Lemasters, G.: Development and evaluation of a microprocessor-based ergonomic dosimeter for evaluating carpentry tasks. Appl. Ergon. **30**(6), 543–553 (1999)
10. Bootsman, R., Markopoulos, P., Qi, Q., Wang, Q., Timmermans, A.A.: Wearable technology for posture monitoring at the workplace. Int. J. Hum Comput Stud. **132**, 99–111 (2019)
11. Calvo-Gutiérrez, J., et al.: Inter-rater reliability of clinical mobility measures in ankylosing spondylitis. BMC Musculoskelet. Disord. **17**(1), 1–6 (2016)
12. Carbonaro, N., et al.: A wearable sensor-based platform for surgeon posture monitoring: a tool to prevent musculoskeletal disorders. Int. J. Environ. Res. Public Health **18**(7), 3734 (2021)
13. Carney, D.R., Cuddy, A.J., Yap, A.J.: Power posing: brief nonverbal displays affect neuroendocrine levels and risk tolerance. Psychol. Sci. **21**(10), 1363–1368 (2010)
14. Caviedes, J.E., Li, B., Jammula, V.C.: Wearable sensor array design for spine posture monitoring during exercise incorporating biofeedback. IEEE Trans. Biomed. Eng. **67**(10), 2828–2838 (2020)
15. Char, D.S., Shah, N.H., Magnus, D.: Implementing machine learning in health care-addressing ethical challenges. N. Engl. J. Med. **378**(11), 981 (2018)
16. Charness, N., Dijkstra, K., Jastrzembski, T., Weaver, S., Champion, M.: Are laptop computers a health risk for an aging population? Gerontechnol. Int. J. Fundament. Aspects Technol. Serve Ageing Soc. **9**, 415–420 (2010)
17. Clever, H.M., Erickson, Z., Kapusta, A., Turk, G., Liu, K., Kemp, C.C.: Bodies at rest: 3d human pose and shape estimation from a pressure image using synthetic data. In: Proceedings of the IEEE/CVF Conference on Computer Vision and Pattern Recognition, pp. 6215–6224 (2020)
18. Conforti, I., Mileti, I., Del Prete, Z., Palermo, E.: Measuring biomechanical risk in lifting load tasks through wearable system and machine-learning approach. Sensors **20**(6), 1557 (2020)
19. Fathi, A., Curran, K.: Detection of spine curvature using wireless sensors. J. King Saud. Univ. Sci. **29**(4), 553–560 (2017)
20. Fürst, M., Gupta, S.T., Schuster, R., Wasenmüller, O., Stricker, D.: HPERL: 3D human pose estimation from RGB and lidar. In: 2020 25th International Conference on Pattern Recognition (ICPR), pp. 7321–7327. IEEE (2021)
21. Garrido-Castro, J.L., et al.: Validation of a new objective index to measure spinal mobility: the University of Cordoba Ankylosing Spondylitis Metrology Index (UCOASMI). Rheumatol. Int. **34**(3), 401–406 (2014)
22. Gianino, J.M., Paice, J.A., York, M.M.: Spinal cord anatomy. In: Intrathecal Drug Therapy for Spasticity and Pain, pp. 3–14 (1996)
23. Gleadhill, S., Lee, J.B., James, D.: The development and validation of using inertial sensors to monitor postural change in resistance exercise. J. Biomech. **49**(7), 1259–1263 (2016)
24. Gopalai, A., Senanayake, S.A., Lim, K.H.: Intelligent vibrotactile biofeedback system for real-time postural correction on perturbed surfaces. In: 2012 12th International Conference on Intelligent Systems Design and Applications (ISDA), pp. 973–978. IEEE (2012)
25. Hachaj, T., Ogiela, M.R.: Rule-based approach to recognizing human body poses and gestures in real time. Multimedia Syst. **20**(1), 81–99 (2014)

26. Hamilton, N.P.: Kinesiology: Scientific Basis of Human Motion. Brown & Benchmark (2011)
27. Hansraj, K.K.: Assessment of stresses in the cervical spine caused by posture and position of the head. Surg Technol Int **25**(25), 277–9 (2014)
28. Huang, L., Galinsky, A.D., Gruenfeld, D.H., Guillory, L.E.: Powerful postures versus powerful roles: which is the proximate correlate of thought and behavior? Psychol. Sci. **22**(1), 95–102 (2011)
29. Intolo, P., Carman, A.B., Milosavljevic, S., Abbott, J.H., Baxter, G.D.: The spineangel®: examining the validity and reliability of a novel clinical device for monitoring trunk motion. Man. Ther. **15**(2), 160–166 (2010)
30. Jordan, M.I., Mitchell, T.M.: Machine learning: trends, perspectives, and prospects. Science **349**(6245), 255–260 (2015). https://doi.org/10.1126/science.aaa8415
31. Klatt, B., et al.: A conceptual framework for the progression of balance exercises in persons with balance and vestibular disorders. Phys. Med. Rehabilit. Int. **2**(4) (2015)
32. Kuo, Y.L., Huang, K.Y., Kao, C.Y., Tsai, Y.J.: Sitting posture during prolonged computer typing with and without a wearable biofeedback sensor. Int. J. Environ. Res. Public Health **18**(10), 5430 (2021)
33. Larrea-Araujo, C., Ayala-Granja, J., Vinueza-Cabezas, A., Acosta-Vargas, P.: Ergonomic risk factors of teleworking in Ecuador during the COVID-19 pandemic: a cross-sectional study. Int. J. Environ. Res. Public Health **18**(10), 5063 (2021)
34. Liaqat, S., Dashtipour, K., Arshad, K., Assaleh, K., Ramzan, N.: A hybrid posture detection framework: integrating machine learning and deep neural networks. IEEE Sens. J. **21**(7), 9515–9522 (2021)
35. Lim, C., Basah, S., Ali, M., Fook, C.: Wearable posture identification system for good sitting position. J. Telecommun. Electron. Comput. Eng. **10**(1-16), 135–140 (2018)
36. Lin, J.F., Kulić, D.: Human pose recovery using wireless inertial measurement units. Physiol. Meas. **33**(12), 2099 (2012)
37. Lin, W.Y., Chou, W.C., Tsai, T.H., Lin, C.C., Lee, M.Y.: Development of a wearable instrumented vest for posture monitoring and system usability verification based on the technology acceptance model. Sensors **16**(12), 2172 (2016)
38. Lin, W.Y., Lee, M.Y., Chou, W.C.: The design and development of a wearable posture monitoring vest. In: 2014 IEEE International Conference on Consumer Electronics (ICCE), pp. 329–330. IEEE (2014)
39. Lo Piano, S.: Ethical principles in machine learning and artificial intelligence: cases from the field and possible ways forward (2020). https://www.nature.com/articles/s41599-020-0501-9#citeas
40. Lou, E., Lam, G.C., Hill, D.L., Wong, M.S.: Development of a smart garment to reduce kyphosis during daily living. Med. Biol. Eng. Comput. **50**, 1147–1154 (2012)
41. Lovell, W.W., Winter, R.B., Morrissy, R.T., Weinstein, S.L.: Lovell and Winter's Pediatric Orthopaedics, vol. 1. Lippincott Williams & Wilkins (2006)
42. Lowe, B.D., Weir, P., Andrews, D.: Observation-based posture assessment : review of current practice and recommendations for improvement (2014). https://stacks.cdc.gov/view/cdc/24085 report
43. Madsen, O., Hansen, L., Rytter, A., Suetta, C., Egsmose, C.: The bath metrology index as assessed by a trained and an untrained rater in patients with spondylarthropathy: a study of intra-and inter-rater agreements. Clin. Rheumatol. **28**(1), 35–40 (2009)

44. Marcus, G.: Deep learning: a critical appraisal. arXiv preprint arXiv:1801.00631 (2018)
45. Martindale, J.H., Sutton, C.J., Goodacre, L.: An exploration of the inter-and intra-rater reliability of the bath ankylosing spondylitis metrology index. Clin. Rheumatol. **31**(11), 1627–1631 (2012)
46. Mathis, M.W., Mathis, A.: Deep learning tools for the measurement of animal behavior in neuroscience. Curr. Opin. Neurobiol. **60**, 1–11 (2020)
47. Michaud, F., Lugrís, U., Cuadrado, J.: Determination of the 3d human spine posture from wearable inertial sensors and a multibody model of the spine. Sensors **22**(13), 4796 (2022)
48. Miyajima, S., Tanaka, T., Imamura, Y., Kusaka, T.: Lumbar joint torque estimation based on simplified motion measurement using multiple inertial sensors. In: 2015 37th Annual International Conference of the IEEE Engineering in Medicine and Biology Society (EMBC), pp. 6716–6719. IEEE (2015)
49. Moon, G., Lee, K.M.: Neuralannot: neural annotator for in-the-wild expressive 3d human pose and mesh training sets. arXiv preprint arXiv:2011.11232 (2020)
50. Moon, K.S., Gombatto, S.P., Phan, K., Ozturk, Y.: Extraction of lumbar spine motion using a 3-IMU wearable cluster. Sensors **23**(1), 182 (2023)
51. Moro, A.: Impact of the covid-19 confinement measures on telework in Italy-a qualitative survey. Tech. rep., JRC Working Papers Series on Labour, Education and Technology (2020)
52. Nag, P.K.: Musculoskeletal disorders: office menace. In: Office Buildings. DSI, pp. 105–126. Springer, Singapore (2019). https://doi.org/10.1007/978-981-13-2577-9_4
53. Nath, N.D., Akhavian, R., Behzadan, A.H.: Ergonomic analysis of construction worker's body postures using wearable mobile sensors. Appl. Ergon. **62**, 107–117 (2017)
54. O'Sullivan, K., O'Sullivan, L., Campbell, A., O'Sullivan, P., Dankaerts, W.: Towards monitoring lumbo-pelvic posture in real-life situations: concurrent validity of a novel posture monitor and a traditional laboratory-based motion analysis system. Man. Ther. **17**(1), 77–83 (2012)
55. O'Sullivan, K., Verschueren, S., Pans, S., Smets, D., Dekelver, K., Dankaerts, W.: Validation of a novel spinal posture monitor: comparison with digital video fluoroscopy. Eur. Spine J. **21**, 2633–2639 (2012)
56. O'Sullivan, K., Verschueren, S., Pans, S., Smets, D., Dekelver, K., Dankaerts, W.: Validation of a novel spinal posture monitor: comparison with digital videofluoroscopy. Eur. Spine J. **21**(12), 2633–2639 (2012)
57. Pérez-D'Arpino, C., Shah, J.A.: Fast target prediction of human reaching motion for cooperative human-robot manipulation tasks using time series classification. In: 2015 IEEE International Conference on Robotics and Automation (ICRA), pp. 6175–6182. IEEE (2015)
58. Petropoulos, A., Sikeridis, D., Antonakopoulos, T.: Wearable smart health advisors: an IMU-enabled posture monitor. IEEE Consum. Electron. Mag. **9**(5), 20–27 (2020)
59. Piwek, L., Ellis, D.A., Andrews, S., Joinson, A.: The rise of consumer health wearables: promises and barriers. PLoS Med. **13**(2), e1001953 (2016)
60. Ribeiro, D.C., Milosavljevic, S., Abbott, J.H.: Effectiveness of a lumbopelvic monitor and feedback device to change postural behaviour: a protocol for the elf cluster randomised controlled trial. BMJ Open **7**(1), e015568 (2017)
61. Ribeiro, D.C., Sole, G., Abbott, J.H., Milosavljevic, S.: The effectiveness of a lumbopelvic monitor and feedback device to change postural behavior: a feasibility randomized controlled trial. J. Orthop. Sports Phys. Therapy **44**(9), 702–711 (2014)

62. Samiei-Zonouz, R., Memarzadeh-Tehran, H., Rahmani, R.: Smartphone-centric human posture monitoring system. In: 2014 IEEE Canada International Humanitarian Technology Conference-(IHTC), pp. 1–4. IEEE (2014)
63. Sardini, E., Serpelloni, M., Pasqui, V.: Daylong sitting posture measurement with a new wearable system for at home body movement monitoring. In: 2015 IEEE International Instrumentation and Measurement Technology Conference (I2MTC) Proceedings, pp. 652–657. IEEE (2015)
64. Sardini, E., Serpelloni, M., Pasqui, V.: Daylong sitting posture measurement with a new wearable system for at home body movement monitoring. In: 2015 IEEE International Instrumentation and Measurement Technology Conference (I2MTC) Proceedings, pp. 652–657. IEEE (2015)
65. Six Dijkstra, M.W., et al.: Ethical considerations of using machine learning for decision support in occupational health: an example involving periodic workers' health assessments. J. Occup. Rehabil. **30**(3), 343–353 (2020)
66. Stollenwerk, K., Müller, J., Hinkenjann, A., Krüger, B.: Analyzing spinal shape changes during posture training using a wearable device. Sensors **19**(16), 3625 (2019)
67. Tsuchiya, Y., et al.:: Calibration method for lumbosacral dimensions in wearable sensor system of lumbar alignment. In: 2015 37th Annual International Conference of the IEEE Engineering in Medicine and Biology Society (EMBC), pp. 3909–3912. IEEE (2015)
68. Tsuchiya, Y., et al.: Calibration method for lumbosacral dimensions in wearable sensor system of lumbar alignment. In: 2015 37th Annual International Conference of the IEEE Engineering in Medicine and Biology Society (EMBC), pp. 3909–3912. IEEE (2015)
69. Tsuchiya, Y., Matsuo, Y., Tanaka, T.: Estimation of lumbar load by 2d reconstruction of spine line using wearable sensor system. In: 2014 IEEE International Conference on Systems, Man, and Cybernetics (SMC), pp. 3669–3674. IEEE (2014)
70. Valdivia, S., Blanco, R., Uribe, A., Penuela, L., Rojas, D., Kapralos, B.: A spinal column exergame for occupational health purposes. In: GALA 2017, pp. 83–92. Springer, Heidelberg (2017)
71. Voinea, G.D., Butnariu, S., Mogan, G.: Measurement and geometric modelling of human spine posture for medical rehabilitation purposes using a wearable monitoring system based on inertial sensors. Sensors **17**(1), 3 (2016)
72. Walsh, J., Eccleston, C., Keogh, E.: Pain communication through body posture: the development and validation of a stimulus set. Pain **155**(11), 2282–2290 (2014). https://doi.org/10.1016/j.pain.2014.08.019
73. Wang, Z., et al.: Using wearable sensors to capture posture of the human lumbar spine in competitive swimming. IEEE Trans. Hum. Mach. Syst. **49**(2), 194–205 (2019)
74. Wielgos, S., Dolezalek, E., Min, C.H.: Garment integrated spinal posture detection using wearable magnetic sensors. In: 2020 42nd Annual International Conference of the IEEE Engineering in Medicine and Biology Society (EMBC), pp. 4030–4033. IEEE (2020)
75. Winter, D., MacKinnon, C., Ruder, G., Wieman, C.: An integrated EMG/biomechanical model of upper body balance and posture during human gait. Prog. Brain Res. **97**, 359–367 (1993)
76. Wu, W.S., Lin, W.Y., Lee, M.Y.: Forward-flexed posture detection for the early Parkinson's disease symptom. In: 2014 IEEE International Conference on Systems, Man, and Cybernetics (SMC), pp. 1181–1185. IEEE (2014)

77. Wu, Y., Chen, K., Fu, C.: Natural gesture modeling and recognition approach based on joint movements and arm orientations. IEEE Sens. J. **16**(21), 7753–7761 (2016)
78. Xu, J., et al.: Configurable, wearable sensing and vibrotactile feedback system for real-time postural balance and gait training: proof-of-concept. J. Neuroeng. Rehabil. **14**, 1–10 (2017)

Role of Big Data, AI and Deep Learning in Medical Image Training Models and Decision Support System Using I4.0 Technologies

Kavita Bhatt[✉] and S. Mohan Kumar

School of Engineering and Technology, CMR University, Bangalore 560037, India
kavitabhattphd@gmail.com

Abstract. The area of diagnostic decision assistance in radiology is going through a rapid shift with the availability of a lot of patient information and the advancement of new AI (Artificial Intelligence) techniques of ML (Machine Learning), like DL (Deep Learning). They have the potential to offer imaging professionals tools that will increase the precision and effectiveness of diagnosis and therapy. This paper will discuss the development of the area of radiology and general trends emphasizing advancements in diagnostic decision assistance from the earliest rule-based expert systems to contemporary cognitive assistants utilizing I4.0 technology. The accuracy, dependability, and productivity of electronic equipment in the healthcare industry must be improved with the use of the IoMT (Internet of Medical Things). Researchers are building a digital healthcare system by connecting the already available medical resources and healthcare services. Although IoT is converging across many disciplines, our attention is on the scientific contributions of IoT in the healthcare domain.

In terms of medical services in healthcare, this article discusses IoT applications, user contributions, and upcoming problems specifically in medical imaging hence the name Internet of Medical Imaging Things. It also gives a complete overview of the latest developments of ML approaches broadly utilized for Medical Imaging Diagnostic using I4.0 by classifying the study as per the ML methods, equipment, and machinery used and a foundation for future research.

Keywords: Artificial intelligence · medical image datasets · Image storage · Image quality assessment · diagnostic decision support · artificial intelligence · cognitive assistants · deep learning · knowledge and reasoning · diagnostic decision support · cognitive assistants · deep learning · knowledge and reasoning · machine learning · medical image analysis

1 Introduction

Medical image analysis yields vital information to clinicians, and radiologists to interpret, predict, and diagnose disease. There are various modalities available like X-Ray, Mammography, CT scan, etc. through which the disease is diagnosed. There are various techniques and methods available to process and analyze medical imaging sources. With recent disruptions in data science medical image analysis and processing is improving drastically and it has open room to explore various aspects of imaging in different processes like medical image classification, segmentation, reconstruction, enhancement, etc. With the availability of significant patient datasets and deep learning the diagnostic support system using radiology is taking a great transformation leveraging deep learning techniques.

[1] With the rise of AI, radio mics came into being. In radio mics, digital pictures that are usually analyzed by doctors in a "qualitative" way are turned into "quantitative" data. The digital data may then be applied to teach ML methods to detect particular traits that could provide information about a diagnosis or prognosis that is hidden from human sight. Machine learning has driven many advanced solutions in multiple fields like automated translation, self-assisted driving, etc. with the help of natural language processing and computer vision but the health sector is one such field that is still in the exploration stage due to its underlying hazard if not taken care of properly. Accurate prediction is one of the crucial outcomes of image processing and analysis [2].

[3] Professionals have referred to the current state of industries as "The Fourth Industrial Revolution," also recognized as "Industry 4.0" or (I4.0). Industry 4.0 is primarily focused on integrating physical and digital technologies in manufacturing situations [4]. The ability to gather large amounts of operational and process conditions data produced by various types of equipment and use the data to make automated fault detection and diagnosis to reduce downtime, rise component utilization, and extend the components' remaining useful lives is made possible by the digital transformation toward I4.0, computerized control, information methods, as well as communication networks.

[5] Industry 4.0 and its supporting information and communication technologies are dramatically transforming both the services and manufacturing sectors. This is particularly true in the health arena, in which the IoT ("Internet of Things"), Cloud and Fog Computing, as well as Big Data technologies are changing eHealth and its whole ecosystem, therefore advancing Healthcare 4.0 [6]. With I4.0, PHM ("Prognostics and Health Management") has become an inescapable trend in smart manufacturing and industrial big data, providing a trustworthy solution for industrial equipment health status. I4.0 and its core technologies are crucial for enabling industrial systems to become autonomous and, as a result, enabling automated data gathering from industrial components and equipment. Machine learning algorithms can automate fault identification and diagnosis using obtained data. However, choosing the right ML methodologies, data types, data sizes, and tools to use ML in industrial systems is very challenging. The improper PdM method, dataset as well as data size could lead to time loss and inefficient maintenance scheduling.

In this article, we will discuss the I4.0 technologies and how they can be used to provide an end-to-end solution starting from scanning to processing to building and training models using AI, ML, and DL, and how best big data and analytics will come into the picture. And a brief on cyber security to address medical image processing would be covered.

In addition to analyzing the current study implementations showing the efficiency of IoMT advantages to patients and the healthcare system. This structured systematic study aims to detect the critical role of IoMT uses in enhancing healthcare systems. It also provides a summary of the technologies that supplement IoMT and discusses the complications in creating a smart healthcare system. The many layers, their functions, and processes in IoMT are discussed in the first section. The 2nd section describes the many technologies that work along with IoMT to streamline the delivery of healthcare in the current day. IoMT applications in the healthcare industry are covered in the 3rd section. The final section lists the obstacles to the widespread use of IoMT before providing a crisp conclusion to the entire discussion (Fig. 1).

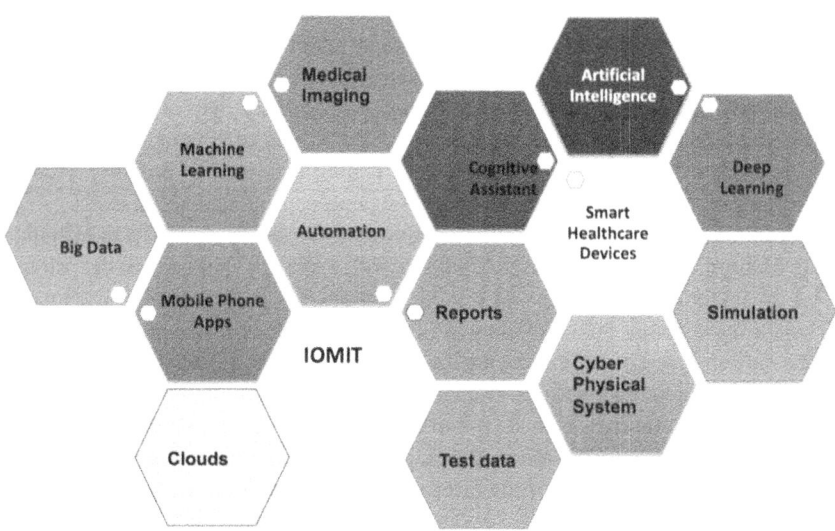

Fig. 1. Anatomy of Internet of Medical Imaging Thing (IOMT)

2 I4.0 Technologies and Habituation of IoMT

[7] The IoT is a system of interconnected physical objects, or "Things," that enable information sharing across systems and devices. Since Ashton first mentioned the IoT)in 1999, there has been an exponential expansion that has produced around 10 billion connected IoT devices now, with a forecast rise to nearly 25 billion by 2025.1,2 In terms of technical implementation, it means expediting data exchange and data storing on a safe cloud server, where a network of linked computer devices may share data and speak with one another through the server. Numerous innovations have been made on items and gadgets to make them "smart" using "embedded software" that either allows new capabilities or updates their present capability.

[5] I4.0 technologies in conjunction with Bigdata, Cyber-Physical systems, Cloud computing, AI, and the Internet of Things can be efficiently leveraged to build a system used in medical imaging and processing. Data can be collected, analyzed, processed, and distributed in a timely fashion. The overall solution can improve the radiology department by providing state-of-the-art solutions providing efficient and intelligent

decision support and virtual accessibility of the evaluation data. With the help of data science technologies like AI, ML, and DL it can be a self-learned model to take efficient decisions on its own and provide targeted solutions, reducing human intervention. The "Internet of Medical Things" (IoMT) is a set of hardware and software for the medical industry that connects to Internet computer networks to access healthcare IT systems. Medical devices with Wi-Fi capabilities provide the machine-to-machine connection at the foundation of IoMT.

IoMT has many applications in the medical field, but remote/self-health monitoring of numerous vital functions, such as nutrition status, movement monitoring, skin temperature, heart rate, general health conditions monitoring, and rehabilitation of infected or elderly patients, are more significant and directly affect life expectancy as well as morbidity and mortality rates. A smart hospital information system was developed where different technologies, such as CT and MRI scans, could be combined with lab data to enable enhanced diagnosis of medical emergencies, supporting medical personnel in monitoring and making the proper treatment decisions. It is noteworthy that by making hospitals "smart," equipment costs may also be decreased since irregularities that can impair the precision of certain readings obtained from medical devices may be discovered earlier, which would prevent higher maintenance expenses.

[7] The adoption of IoMT and associated technologies have addressed several issues using sensors, robotics, telemedicine, remote monitoring, etc. However, widespread adoption is challenging for many reasons, including data security and privacy concerns, huge data management, scalability, and upgradeability. Although a great deal of data has already been collected and disseminated, this systematic review will help doctors, researchers, policymakers, and others determine the value of IoMT in healthcare [7]. The health of an unprecedented number of patients must be closely monitored during the pre-and post-infection phases of the current COVID-19 epidemic. Telehealth has

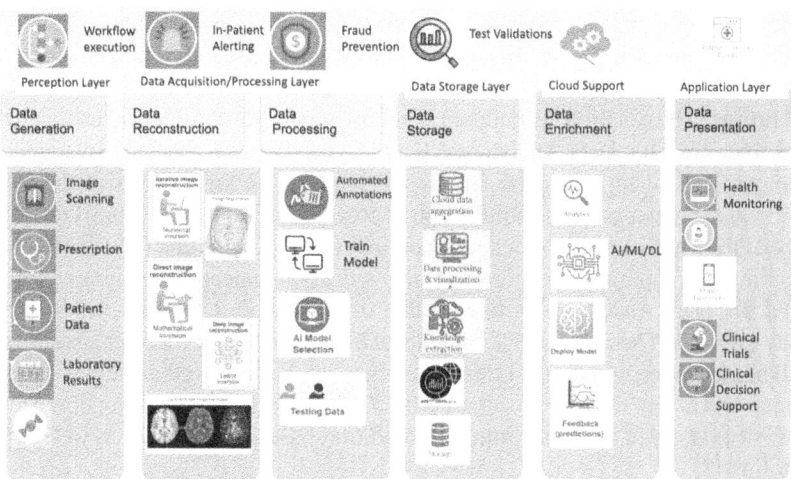

Fig. 2. Different Layers of IoMT(specific to Medical Imaging). Image references from [15, 19–21]

been utilized successfully for remote patient monitoring, screening, and treatment by both caregivers or healthcare practitioners and patients. Smart gadgets powered by the IoMT are proliferating everywhere, especially during a worldwide epidemic. Healthcare, however, is seen as being one of IoMT's most difficult application sectors due to the large quantity of demand.

Figure 2 depicts the different layers of IoMT which are detailed out in later section.

3 Existing Solution and Problem

Many improvements have been made with the use of computer-assisted software and deep learning, but concerns with the shortage of training data, particularly labelled data, are still often addressed in the medical imaging community and have a negative influence on how medical image processing is carried out in general. To increase the overall effectiveness of medical image analysis and subsequent diagnosis, data augmentation techniques using data science and deep learning models are put to use. However, these techniques frequently run into problems when data must be interpreted in a connected environment where data sets must be correlated among various other datasets. To evaluate the vast number of image sources and provide an intelligent and individualized evaluation to the person or health unit, radiologists require a connected yet distributed environment. In addition, picture privacy is a problem that this article does not address. It would be quickly snatched. Big data and deep learning principles are used to analyze data, and a change in one dataset may be used to identify the necessary association and alter the image of a linked dataset that is related to it.

[1] Another industry leader, GE Healthcare, has its Effortless Workflow model that similarly offers users AI-based tools to automate and simplify time-consuming tasks. Prior to scanning, the applications use machine learning to automatically suggest protocols for each exam, position patients in the scanner, provide the correct scan range for head, chest, abdomen, and pelvis scans, including multigroup scans. Post scanning, the tools help with image review and analysis on a Revolution Ascend computed tomography (CT) scanner.

Solution: The solution to building a robust model to do efficient medical imaging involves big data, Data Analytics, AI, and Cyber-Physical Systems leveraging I4.0 technologies and their landscape. Below are some of the key aspects of the solution [3]. I4.0, also known as the Fourth Industrial Revolution, is primarily powered by CPS ("Cyber-Physical System"), which relies on IoT, Cloud Computing (which offers virtually unlimited computing, and storage, along with communication resources as utilities, such as Big Data Analytics (to derive value from difficult data sets); and on-demand and pay-per-use). These enormous amounts of data gathered for ML contain a wealth of valuable knowledge and useful information that can boost the efficiency of all system dynamics and manufacturing processes. These data can also be used to support decision-making in a variety of contexts, primarily condition-based maintenance as well as health monitoring [8].

4 Demystifying IOMIT – and C's of Big Data and AI Role in Building Models and Connected Network

[8] Radiologists are starting to wonder whether ML, artificial intelligence, and its utilization of big data would eventually result in machines taking the place of radiologists in light of recent research showing accuracy levels higher as compared to clinician-grade in reading imaging in a small number of specialties. Although the discipline will continue to develop, replacing radiologists is a considerably more difficult prospect when taken into account commonly across the field, where a vast number of variants of modalities, modes, views, anatomical variances, and disease symptoms are required to be addressed. An attempt is being made by a new generation of robots to complement radiologists' decision-making rather than replace them by pre-analyzing the data and providing suggestions. Cognitive assistants are those devices that collaborate with medical professionals like radiologists and cardiologists. Recent studies have demonstrated that these devices have a higher likelihood of being incorporated into clinical workflows by doctors than those that aim to completely replace professionals.

Big data is known for its very infamous 6 C's which are Connection, Cloud, Cyber, Content, Community, and Customization. With the help of these C's a robust model can be generated to have effective medical imaging and scanning procedures and provide an efficient diagnosis in return.

The connection ensures data from multiple modalities are networked and well connected to integrate and transfer data in different entities of the health unit.

Cloud keeps the data in a distributed and remote server and provides data on a need basis to the health unit.

The cyber-physical system ensures there is needed computing power enabled to process large queries aligned to image processing. To have such large processing big data is paramount.

Content: Medical imaging system needs a huge amount of medical data to build and train models and to save the real analysis data. The DICOM ("Digital Imaging and Communications in Medicine") datasets are referred to here. To have a better diagnosis in place, usually, this content is searched.

Community: Data distribution and availability for future research and contributing to the wider dataset are very important in the medical imaging field. With the help of I4.0 technologies data can be diagnosed, mapped efficiently, and distributed to multiple parties of interest.

Customization: A practitioner often deals with interpretation and its evaluation. A robust system is in place to aid multiple query-based diagnoses and have an algorithm in place to provide intended customization for clinical processing and to foster personalized assessment and evaluation.

On the other hand, AI leverages huge amounts of data to build its model which further leverages ML and DL techniques. With the help of DL and AI techniques, medical image data can be predicted. But to scale the solution a large amount of data set can be processed using Bigdata, processed, predicted, and transferred to different departments in no time and thus enhancing the overall efficiency of the diagnosis and prediction.

A typical Model: It can be clubbed as an **e-System or Smart Health** but focuses mainly on **medical Imaging processing** and privacy/security. Figure 3 below proposes a high-level anatomy of the proposal and solution using I4.0 and IoMT technologies leveraging big data, cloud, security, and benefits of advanced ML and DL methods.

Large volumes of patient data from ML and clinical expertise are both used to power cognitive assistants. In our research group, a new breed of clinical decision support machines is being developed.

We tackle the diagnostic decision support problem by implying tools and techniques of IoT, I4.O, and IoMT.

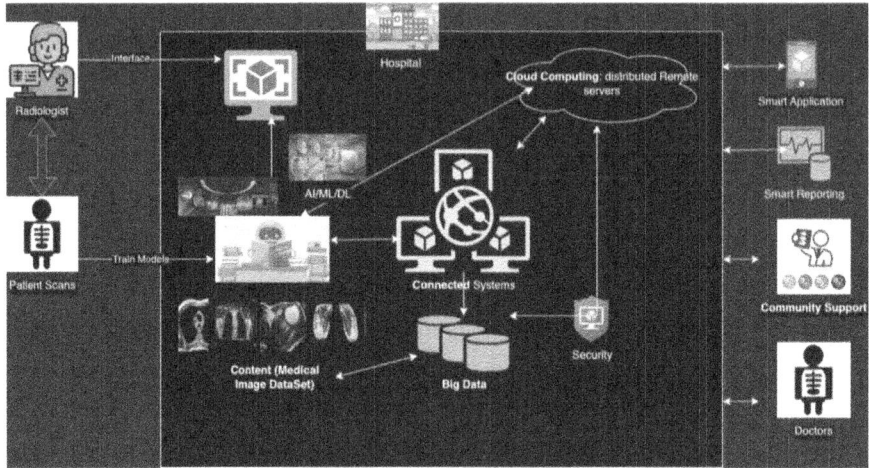

Fig. 3. A typical Diagnostic Support System for Medical Imaging - IOMIT

4.1 Stage 1 Data Preparation/ Scanning

[9] One of the most well-known options is AI, which has the potential to completely transform both clinical practice and medical research. The correct preparation of the medical pictures to be utilized by the AI-driven solutions is the cornerstone enabling the creation of dependable and robust AI algorithms. Here, we offer a thorough overview of the procedures that must be followed to prepare medical photos before creating or using AI algorithms. The first patient anatomical structure is scanned per the doctor's advice and the radiologist records that data and feeds it to the system where with the help of AI/ML technologies data is classified, segmented, augmented, and in parallel the data is fed to the data set and image data set for further training purpose and bringing up the robust data model to perform supervised or unsupervised learning techniques to diagnose the issue.

A typical medical picture preparation pipeline involves the following basic steps:
- image acquisition at clinical sites,
- image de-identification to protect patient privacy and erase identifying information,

- data filtration to ensure the quality of the images and related information,
- image storage, and
- image annotation.

4.2 Stage 2 Image Reconstruction Using AI/ML Techniques

The 2nd significant area that benefits from the application of AI is post-scanning picture reconstruction. Finally, depending on variations from how they normally appear, we search for abnormalities in chosen anatomical locations [10]. Numerous machine learning techniques, including support vector machine variations, random forests, and deep learning networks, are used to train machines using massive clinician-annotated data sets. Once the anomalous parts have been identified, cognitive assistants look through other clinical data sources, especially text data, to uncover other details that may be used as clinical characteristics.

As signal-to-noise ratios increase, scan times decrease, diagnostic confidence increases, and workflow is sped up. For this reason, deep-learning techniques are widely utilized to enhance picture reconstruction when applying AI.

4.3 Stage 3 Image Reading and Interpretation

[11] In the reading and interpretation of the images, the 3rd main use of AI in radiology, third parties, frequently start-ups, do become involved. Radiologists read a significant volume of images every day. Finding anything alarming without noting false positives might be challenging; "clinical decision" support based on AI can be helpful.

George et al. in [11] the digital images prepared in the widespread DICOM format are accessed by the radiologists using the PACS ("Picture Archiving Communication System"). Due to the standardization of these pictures and the PACS, it is less complicated for other parties to utilize the information when creating algorithms. Since the algorithms can be applied regardless of the camera used to take the picture, they may then make them available to the largest user base possible. It was predicted that the market for AI within medical imaging will reach $1.06 billion in 2021 and grow at an average annual rate of 45.7% to $10.14 billion by 2027.2 These companies are developing a wide range of image interpretation tools for X-ray, CT, ultrasound, and MRI images in addition to MRI. There are several potential applications for these tools.

4.4 Stage 4 Data Processing:

Image preparation tools are an important part of creating and using AI solutions. Big data may be used by AI to create a fine-tuned modal. Additionally, AI may assist large data in decision-making and assessment. The gathered patient clinical data is then contrasted with a substantial body of clinical knowledge that has previously been weighted by patient-related statistics obtained via "electronic health record" analysis. Declarative as well as procedural information is utilized to draw new findings about suggestions for diagnosis, and therapy, such as the next-best test, and forecasting results related to the results.

Multimodal clinical reasoning using learned distributions from massive patient data sets is an efficient inference engine for clinical decision assistance in a cognitive assistant system. The information is subsequently sent to several other linked systems after being stored on the cloud [9]. With the help of cloud computing the data is stored, transported, and interacted with smart devices for further diagnosis, training the data model leveraging AL/ML and big data queries.

4.5 Application/Service Layer

This is the abstract layer that can be leveraged in the form of an application user interface for final diagnosis and reporting purposes.

The application layer's main function is to provide application-specific services and to understand data. The application layer uses AI and DL learning to interpret the EMR data and monitor changes and patterns in the data for use in making diagnostic and therapeutic choices (contextualization of data).

In addition to language processing, text recognition, and image analysis other scientific uses include those linked to health care, like malignant tumors, benign, Alzheimer's disease, cardiac arrhythmia, bone disease, prognostication of congestive heart failure, diabetes and mental health management, medical outcomes, designing of drug activity, risk, and gene mutation expression prediction.

5 Findings and Challenges

[14] The biggest challenge in this discipline is still acquiring a sizable number of precise classifications for imaging tests and their abnormal regions from clinical professionals, despite the tremendous developments in DL and reasoning approaches in cognitive assistants. It is now possible to find web-based annotation tools that are distributed in the cloud and use a crowdsourcing paradigm for physician annotations but scaling up these projects is still difficult. It appears reasonable to employ a priori knowledge of clinically important characteristics for a certain area to bias deep learning systems. Learning from incomplete, incorrect, or ambiguously labeled data is still a current study topic in science. Deep learning approaches start to include a priori clinical information into the process of learning rather than using it afterward via reasoning algorithms as cognitive components of learning grow more important.

Established academics have also drawn attention to such higher-layer semantic DL networks. Last but not least, investigators are starting to doubt the existing method of creating DL networks task by task and are thinking about creating enormous DL networks that can simultaneously resolve the issues of viewpoint recognition, anatomy segmentation, anomaly detection, and other problems all in one network. The field wants to provide semi-automatic ground truth labelling techniques more quickly. In these techniques, a computer learns patterns from a smaller number of annotations provided by clinicians utilizing active learning models. Research on deep learning networks also needs to advance. While DL may automatically learn characteristics through the process of corrective learning, researchers are beginning to wonder if it is appropriate to utilize networks with this many layers that take so long to converge.

Commercial uses of such technologies are starting to emerge in a range of use cases where machines might be helpful as academics continue to overcome the technical obstacles in establishing practical strategies to use big data in medical imaging. Discrepancy identification in patient data, comparing with earlier exams and recording variations, work list priority for brain bleed patients, and semi-automatic report production are a few examples. Another difficult hurdle is the smooth integration of these technologies into clinical workflow.

The risk of exposure is greatly increased when the IoMT data are added to the already existing pool of clinically pertinent medical data.

- Software implementation of analytical methods used in medicine.
- Clinicians must receive training to use apps and the IoMT system efficiently.
- A problem while creating IoMT systems is interoperability to link devices from various suppliers.
- Data breaches are more likely when more devices are connected to other systems and one another.

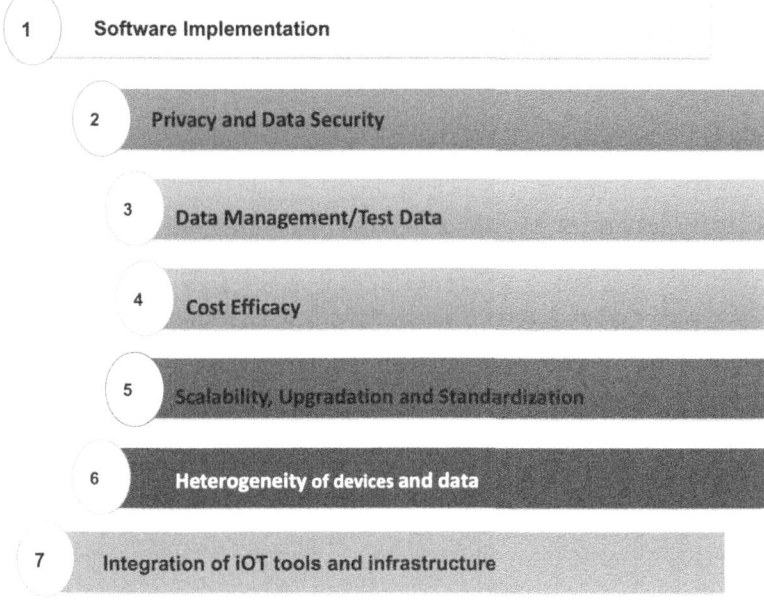

Fig. 4. Challenges of IOMT

Figure 4 highlights the different challenges of IoMT which are detailed out in below section.

Software Implementation: The machine learning and deep learning-driven algorithm and their integration need extensive testing in conjunction with the rest of the ecosystem. It requires experts to develop such software which sometimes is lacking due to lack of the right skillset [12].

Privacy and Data Security: [10, 13, 14] One of the prominent issues in the Internet of Medical Imaging thing is cyber safety and securing large amounts of sensitive health data, especially during transportation.

A lightweight block encryption technique for remote health monitoring was created by the author in [15], with considerations for health security and medical data in an environment of IoMT on the basis of the cloud.

Data management is the capacity to integrate, access, manage, and regulate the flow of data information. Data filtering approaches, including data privacy, data integration, as well as synchronization, are applied to give just application-useful information and conceal extraneous aspects [12].

Scalability/upgradation: [7] Scalability is the capacity of medical equipment to alter in response to environmental changes. Thus, a highly scalable system keeps consistency across the linked devices and may operate effectively using the resources at hand without experiencing any lag. A highly scalable system continues to be more functional in the present as well as future. The requirement for routine upgrading of the current device has increased due to the IoMT technology's ongoing development and developments. This is still challenging in the current fast-paced environment.

[16] Numerous manufacturers and vendors in the healthcare industry mass-produce IoMT-based devices depending on data aggregation, gateway interfaces, and communication protocols, and all claim to have followed established standards and conventions in the development of the product. The use of the appropriate organizations or authorities, like the IETF ("Information Technology and Innovation Foundation"), the ETSI ("European Telecommunications Standards Institute"), and IPSO Internet ("Protocol for Smart Objects") is required for such validation and standardization.

Additionally, EMR recording IoMT devices require validation. Collaboration between scholars, different organizations, and standardizing agencies can make this happen. IoMT devices are not being adopted quickly or widely because of regulatory obstacles including the HITECH ("Health Information Technology for Economic and Clinical Health") Act, HIPAA ("Health Insurance Portability and Accountability Act") compliance, and GDPR ("General Data Protection Regulation").

Heterogeneity of devices and data: [16] Distinct industries have different standards that support their applications. Furthermore, the extent of utilization is limited by the diversity of devices and data from diverse sources, mostly because of inter-operator differences. Interoperability is complicated by the difficulty of exchanging data amongst IoMT systems that have widely varying capabilities. Therefore, developing standardized interfaces is crucial, especially for applications that allow for interoperability across different organizations. Managing the connected devices in an interoperable manner while adopting energy limits is still a key challenge in the IoMT world, where a high volume of data is generated due to the flow of various types of information.

Integration of IoT tools/Infrastructure: [12, 17, 18] Specific to Covid 19 times, financial hardship has increased to encompass numerous people, businesses, and even organizations, restricting the widespread use of IoMT. Cost-effectiveness thus emerges as a major issue that needs proper consideration. IoMT system development, installation, and usage costs must be reasonable. There are several connected sensors and components of medical equipment in the IoMT-based system. Both the manufacturer and the customer are impacted by the cost of upgrading and maintaining these. To stimulate the development of more IoMT devices and make them utilized more frequently, adding sensors with low setup costs and low maintenance needs would be beneficial.

6 Conclusion

The evolution of diagnostic clinical decision assistance in radiology is being aided by big data and ML. We have concentrated on three key elements in this article to provide significant clinical decision support: (1) modelling the radiologist's diagnostic procedure and applying DL to methodically solve important image identification issues (2) using clinical expertise, and (3) integrating clinical inference and reasoning by combining imaging & clinical data with clinical expertise. Although there are still several obstacles to building usable systems that address a broad range of illnesses, the technology is rapidly advancing. The latest in a line of cognitive assistant machines, and clinical decision support systems, presents a novel opportunity for machines to help radiologists and cardiologists perform more effectively. With these kinds of improvements, it won't be long before cognitive clinical assistants are used in every day clinical processes.

Our research is also intended to assist scholars and practitioners in the area in comprehending the enormous potential of IoT in the medical domain and identifying significant hurdles in IoMT. The researchers will also benefit from this effort in their understanding of IoT applications in the healthcare industry.

Acknowledgment. We thank the Directorate of Research and Innovation (DORI) CMR University for training and support. The research is funded by the CMRU student research & innovation fund.

References

1. Cowen, L.: Inside precision medicine. https://www.insideprecisionmedicine.com/artificial-intelligence/how-artificial-intelligence-is-driving-changes-in-radiology/
2. Rana, M., Bhushan, M.: Machine learning and deep learning approach for medical image analysis: diagnosis to detection. Multimedia Tools and Applications (2022)
3. Bhatt, K., Kumar, S.M.: Reindustrialization using industry 4.0 maturity models in msmes and tenets of digital transformation phases. In: 2022 Fourth International Conference on Emerging Research in Electronics, Computer Science and Technology (ICERECT), pp. 1–6 (2022)
4. Çınar, Z.M., Abdussalam Nuhu, A., Qasim, Z., Korhan, O., Mohammed, A., Safaei, B.: Machine learning in predictive maintenance towards sustainable smart manufacturing in industry 4.0}. Sustainability **12**(19) (2020)
5. Aceto, G., Persico, V., Pescapé, A.: Industry 4.0 and health: internet of things, big data, and cloud computing for healthcare 4.0. J. Ind. Inf. Integr. **18**, 100129 (2020)
6. Cinar, Z.M., Zeeshan, Q., Solyali, D.K.O.: Simulation of factory 4.0: a review. In: Industrial Engineering in the Digital Disruption Era: Selected papers from the Global Joint Conference on Industrial Engineering and Its Application Areas, Gazimagusa, North Cyprus, Turkey, GJCIE 2019, pp. 204–216 (2019)

7. Dwivedi, R., Mehrotra, D., Chandra, S.: Potential of internet of medical things (IoMT) applications in building a smart healthcare system: a systematic review. J. Oral Biology and Craniofacial Res. **12**(2), 302–318 (2022)
8. Syeda-Mahmood, T.: Role of big data and machine learning in diagnostic decision support in radiology. J. American College of Radiology **15**(3) (2018)
9. Lekadir, O.D., et al.: Data preparation for artificial intelligence in medical imaging: a comprehensive guide to open-access platforms and tools. Physica Medica **32**, 25–37 (2021)
10. Tsoutsouras, V., Azariadi, D., Koliogewrgi, K., Xydis, S., Soudris, D.: Tsoutsouras, Vasileios and Azariadi, Dimitra and Koliogewrgi, Konstantina and Xydis, Sotirios and Soudris, DimitriosSoftware design and optimization of ECG signals analysis and diagnosis for embedded IoT devices. Components and Services for IoT Platforms pp. 299–322 (2017)
11. Kagadis, G., et al.: Medical imaging displays and their use in image interpretation. Radiographics **33**(1), 275–290 (2013)
12. Pritika, B.S., Azam, S.: A perspective roadmap for IoMT-based early detection and care of the neural disorder, dementia. Advanced Computational Intelligence Technology in Healthcare Management (2021)
13. Stepanian, R.S.H., Sungoor, A., Faisal, A., Philip, N.: Internet of M-Health things 'm-IOT, IET, pp. 1–3 (2011)
14. Bharati, S., Podder, P.: Machine and deep learning for IoT security and privacy: applications, challenges, and future directions. Institute of Information and Communication Technology (IICT)
15. Wang, G., Ye, J.C., De Man, B.: Deep learning for tomographic image reconstruction. Nature Machine Intelligence volume **2**(12), 737–748 (2020)
16. Pritika, B.S., Azam, S.: Risk assessment of heterogeneous IoMT devices: a review. Technologies **11**(1) (2023)
17. embs. IoMT (Internet of Medical Things): Reducing Cost While Improving Patient Care (2020). https://www.embs.org/pulse/articles/iomt-internet-of-medical-things-reducing-cost-while-improving-patient-care/
18. Gulraiz, R., Joyia, J., Liaqat, M., Farooq, A., Rehman, S.: Internet of medical things (IOMT): applications, benefits and future challenges in healthcare domain. Journal of Communications **12** (2017)
19. mri-beyond-segmentation. Deep learning in MRI beyond segmentation: Medical image reconstruction, registration, and synthesis (2020). https://theaisummer.com/mri-beyond-segmentation/
20. Hameed, B., et al.: Engineering and clinical use of artificial intelligence (AI) with machine learning and data science advancements: radiology leading the way for future. Therapeutic Advances in Urology **13** (2021)
21. iomt, 09 March 2020. https://hoornebert.be/tag/iomt/

Generating Breathing Patterns in Real-Time: Low-Latency Respiratory Phase Tracking From 25 Hz PPG

Ian Karman, Yue Sun, Rahil Soroushmojdehi, Jose A. Silva, and Mostafa 'Neo' Mohsenvand(✉)

BrainCo Inc., Somerville, MA, USA
{ian.karman,yue.sun,rahil.soroushmojdehi,jose.silva,
neo.mohsenvand}@brainco.tech

Abstract. This study presents a low-latency, real-time breathing cycle tracking system utilizing a conditional Generative Adversarial Network (GAN) with Wasserstein loss, with a low-powered, low sample rate Photoplethysmography (PPG) sensor. The aim is to provide a clinically accurate respiratory tool capable of tracking and visualizing the breathing cycle and rate in real-time for at-home and general ambulatory applications. To detect breathing activity in real-time, we used a wearable headband with a 25 Hz PPG sensor and an inductive respiratory sensor as ground truth. To meet the real-time and low latency constraints, the inputs were processed in 1-s windows. Signal processing and machine learning techniques were explored, and the proposed GAN-based method with Wasserstein loss and gradient penalty, outperformed others in accurately tracking the ground-truth breathing curve. Leveraging the GAN-generated breathing curve, a peak-detection algorithm calculated the respiratory rate (RR) with an average mean absolute error (MAE) of 1.47 breaths per minute (bpm) across 10 test subjects, comparable to high-sampling rate PPG literature (1 bpm), but with the advantage of 5 times faster real-time monitoring. The GAN-generated respiratory signal from a low-sampling rate wearable PPG sensor demonstrates potential as a viable alternative to traditional respiratory monitoring systems. This system offers valuable breathing monitoring, useful in various applications such as pain management.

Keywords: Machine Learning · Respiratory Tracking · Photoplethysmography · Generative Adversarial Networks · Sequence-to-Sequence · Real-Time Monitoring · Low-Latency · Respiratory Rate · Breathing Patterns

---

I. Karman and Y. Sun—These authors contributed equally to this work.

1 Introduction

The monitoring of patients, both in hospital settings and at home, has significantly benefited from the advancements in wearable devices. These devices provide the ability to continuously and non-invasively track various physiological parameters, enabling timely interventions and improving patient care. Among the vital signs, monitoring breathing in real-time plays a crucial role in assessing respiratory function and detecting respiratory abnormalities [24]. Real-time monitoring of breathing using wearable devices plays a vital role in pain management applications, promoting mindful breathing exercises, and offering valuable insights into a patient's respiratory patterns, respiratory rate (RR), and overall respiratory health. These devices allow individuals to track their breathing patterns in real-time, facilitating better pain control techniques and enhancing overall well-being. By providing immediate feedback on breathing cycles, wearable devices enable individuals to engage in mindful breathing exercises, helping to reduce stress, anxiety, and promote relaxation [10,24]. The convenience and mobility offered by these devices make them ideal for at-home use, empowering individuals to take an active role in managing their pain and engaging in mindfulness practices outside of traditional healthcare settings. Real-time breathing monitoring has promising applications beyond healthcare settings, extending its benefits to athletes, swimmers, and singers. Athletes can optimize their breathing patterns for enhanced performance and injury prevention. Swimmers benefit from improved stroke efficiency and breath control, while singers can refine their breath support and vocal projection. These applications empower individuals in various domains to achieve their best performance and elevate their skills [24].

Several previous works have explored the provision of feedback for breathing control, each employing different techniques and technologies [10]. For instance, Breeze is a mobile application that utilizes a smartphone's microphone to continuously detect breathing phases, subsequently triggering a gamified biofeedback-guided breathing training [20,38]. BreatheBuddy, on the other hand, employs the low-power accelerometer in earbuds to generate various breathing biomarkers, including breathing phase, rate, depth, and symmetry [31]. WiRelax stands out as the first non-contact respiratory biofeedback system, which utilizes WiFi to map changes in Channel State Information to the instantaneous breathing state [19]. Tanaka's research focuses on real-time breathing training for individuals with mild cognitive impairment, using a tablet's camera to analyze face blood flow [42]. Additionally, the Breathing-Mentor app combines effective visualization instructions with biofeedback on deep abdominal breathing, leveraging the accelerometers in mobile phones [11]. Furthermore, Prana company utilizes a strap sensor as a wearable platform for training various at-rest breathing exercises, providing live sensor feedback and through a gamified mobile app [30].

Despite the significant progress made in real-time feedback systems for breathing control, none of the mentioned works have utilized the powerful Photoplethysmography (PPG) sensor. The PPG sensor has the capability to record interactions between cardiac, respiratory, and autonomic functions [2]. Numerous research studies have confirmed that PPG signals encompass distinct modulations, including respiratory induced intensity variations (RIIV), respiratory induced amplitude variations (RIAV), and respiratory induced frequency variations (RIFV) [7,17]. Moreover, PPG sensors integrated into wearable devices, like smartwatches, offer convenient and continuous real-time breathing monitoring. With no additional hassle, users can wear these devices and access their respiratory data seamlessly. This portability enables monitoring during various activities, making them beneficial for athletes, swimmers, singers, and anyone interested in tracking their breathing patterns for health and performance improvement. Additionally, PPG sensors offer convenience due to their non-invasive nature, allowing for comfortable and hassle-free measurements. This combination of accessibility, ease of use, and continuous monitoring makes PPG-based systems a valuable tool for various applications.

Many previous applications incorporating the PPG sensor have primarily focused on detecting parameters such as blood oxygen saturation [4,22,34,39], heart rate [22,34], blood pressure [18,22], and respiration rate [17,25,36,39]. Among these studies, Karlen [17] employed a smart fusion technique to estimate RR using high-sampling rate PPG with 1-s window shifts, achieving an average root mean square error (RMSE) of 3 bpm. Park [25] utilized an adaptive lattice notch filter and high-sampling rate PPG to estimate RR, providing updated results every 5 s. In a more recent study by Selvakumar [36], an incremental merge segmentation technique with high sampling rate PPG and 5-s shifting windows resulted in Mean Absolute Error (MAE) of less than 1 bpm, outperforming previous methods. While the aforementioned studies primarily focused on real-time respiratory rate estimation, none of them specifically addressed the tracking of the breathing cycle as a significant variable. Notably, a recent review by Alian [3] introduced the clinical usage of PPG but did not address the monitoring of the breathing cycle. This underscores the existing research gap and highlights the significance of developing innovative approaches that leverage the potential of the PPG sensor to enable comprehensive and real-time monitoring of the breathing cycle.

This study aims to develop and validate a smart, low-power wearable device utilizing reflectance-type PPG that can monitor the breathing process in real-time. Recently, there has been a growing trend towards the utilization of machine learning techniques in real-time processing of biophysiological data [9,32,40,43], despite the prevalence of signal processing methods in previous studies. Machine learning methods offer significant advantages in handling and analyzing biophysiological data in real-time scenarios. In this study, various signal processing and machine learning algorithms were evaluated to extract respiratory information from raw PPG signals. Among these methods, the Empirical Mode Decomposition (EMD) was tested as a baseline. Additionally, a hybrid model combining an autoencoder (AE) and sequence-to-sequence (Seq2Seq) models was explored. Sequence-to-sequence models were considered due to the input and ground-truth signals being from different domains. Furthermore, a conditional Generative Adversarial Network (GAN) with Wasserstein loss was employed to generate real-time breathing curves from PPG signals. The results revealed that the GAN network outperformed the other two methods, showing its potential as an effective and efficient approach for respiratory monitoring using PPG signals. This GAN model has been specifically designed to effectively operate on PPG devices with very low sampling rates, making it adaptable to other PPG devices. The generated breathing signal can be utilized to extract valuable information regarding the breathing process, including parameters such as breathing depth, inhalation and exhalation durations, or any other relevant data based on the specific application requirements. In addition to this, to further enhance the monitoring of breathing, a peak detection algorithm was employed to estimate RR and breathing depth after generating the breathing curve. By employing this approach, the proposed wearable device offers a cost-effective solution for real-time monitoring of the breathing cycle and RR in individuals.

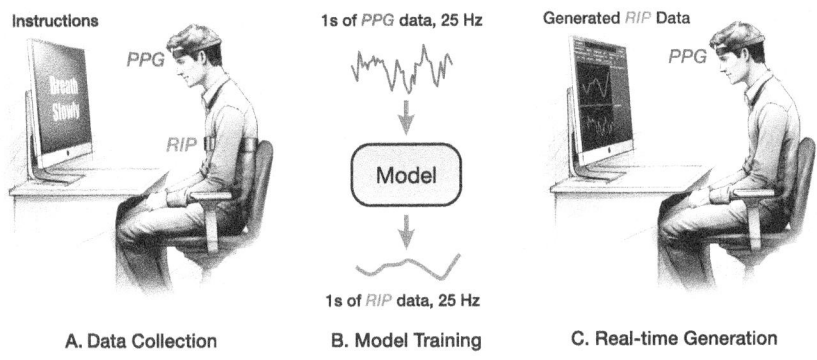

Fig. 1. Overview of the system: A) In data collection, participants are instructed to breathe normally while data from the PPG sensor and Respiratory Inductive Plethysmography (RIP) sensor are recorded. B) Our algorithms, namely Empirical Mode Decomposition (EMD), Sequence-to-Sequence (Seq2Seq), and Generative Adversarial Network (GAN), will be trained utilizing 1-s windows of pre-processed PPG data and RIP signal as input and ground truth, respectively. C) In inference time, respiratory cycle is tracked only using PPG signal and subjects can actively monitor their breathing cycle and respiratory rate (RR) values every 1 s after 20 s of data acquisition.

2 Methods

2.1 Overview

Real-time feedback on breathing phases and respiratory rate holds significant potential for clinical, at-home and general ambulatory applications. However, accurately tracking respiration using a comfortable, low-cost, low-energy platform may pose challenges compared to the precision achieved by devices employed in hospital settings. In this study, we propose an algorithm that leverages a comfortable headband embedded with low-frequency PPG technology.

Figure 1 provides an overview of our system. In the data collection phase, participants are instructed to breathe normally while data from the PPG sensor in the headband and accelerometer data from the chest strap, Respiratory Inductive Plethysmography (RIP) sensor are recorded (Fig. 1A). The 1 s windows of preprocessed PPG data and RIP signal are used as input and ground truth, respectively (Fig. 1B), for the proposed algorithms namely Empirical Mode Decomposition (EMD), Sequence-to-Sequence (Seq2Seq), and Generative Adversarial Network (GAN). The performance of each algorithm in accurately tracking breathing is evaluated, and the output from the most effective algorithm is utilized by the respiration-rate estimator.

During the feedback phase using the trained models (Fig. 1C), subjects can monitor their breathing cycle with a delay of 1 s. Respiratory rate (RR) values are generated after 20 s of data acquisition every 1 s, providing subjects with timely feedback on their respiration.

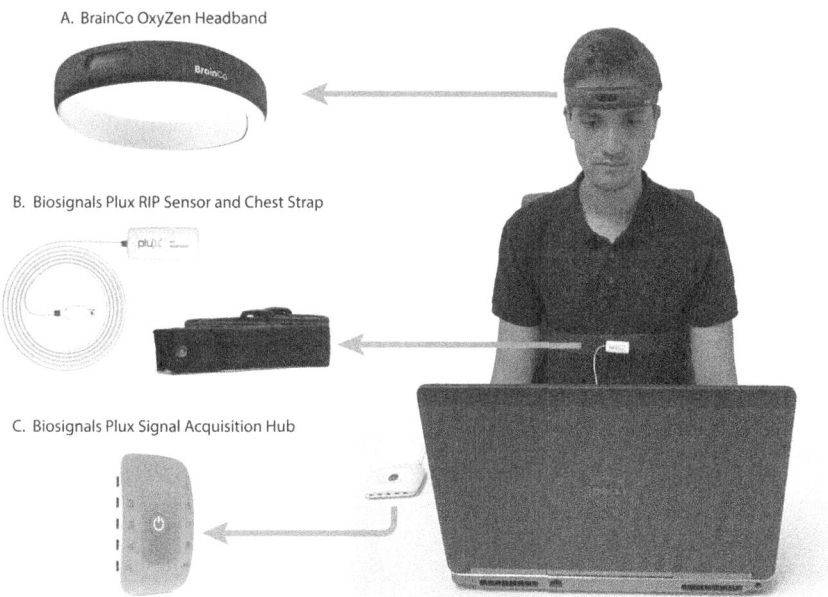

Fig. 2. Experimental setup: Subjects were instructed to breath normally while synchronized data of A) PPG sensor embedded in BrainCo's OxyZen headband and B) Biosignals Plux RIP sensor in conjunction with C) a signal acquisition hub were collected.

2.2 Experimental Setup

For the purpose of this preliminary study, 10 subjects participated (3 females, age 27.4 ± 4.83 years). Participants were instructed to assume a comfortable seated position and breathe normally for 9 min. Figure 2, shows an example of the experimental setup. Subjects participating in the study were instructed to wear a BrainCo's OxyZen headband [8,12], which incorporated a PPG sensor that uses 0.74 mW/s with 25 Hz sampling rate. Additionally, they were instructed to wear a Biosignals Plux RIP sensor [29] with 1000 Hz sampling rate. RIP is a non-invasive technique used to measure respiratory function. The output of the RIP sensor is a continuous waveform that represents the changes in thoracoabdominal dimensions over time, providing valuable information about a person's breathing behavior. All recorded data from PPG and RIP sensor was then transferred to the laptop using bluetooth and all processing was performed using python programming language.

2.3 Pre-processing

We conducted data pre-processing steps to prepare the RIP and PPG data for analysis. The RIP signal, originally acquired at a sampling rate of 1000 Hz, was downsampled to match the sampling rate of the head-worn PPG sensor, which operated at 25 Hz. In order to prepare the inputs and outputs of the models we used a window-based approach, generating 1 s (25 samples) windows of input and output with 20 samples of overlap between hops. Then, we applied a min-max normalization to each 1 s signal of respiratory strap and PPG data.

2.4 Respiratory Signal Generation

EMD. Empirical Mode Decomposition (EMD) is a powerful data analysis method that decomposes a signal into intrinsic mode functions (IMFs) through an iterative sifting process. Each IMF represents a component of the signal with a distinct frequency and timescale [45]. We employed Ensemble EMD (EEMD) which is an improved version of EMD and is previously used in respiratory rate estimation [23,37]. EMD can be sensitive to noise and initial conditions, which may result in variations and inconsistencies in the decomposed IMFs. Ensemble EMD addresses these limitations by introducing an ensemble approach. It involves performing multiple iterations of the EMD process on the same signal with different noise realizations or initial conditions. By averaging or combining the resulting IMFs across iterations, Ensemble EMD aims to improve the overall decomposition quality, reduce artifacts, and enhance the reliability of the extracted components [37]. The key idea behind Ensemble EMD is to leverage the variations introduced by different noise realizations or initial conditions to enhance the robustness of the decomposition.

The use of EEMD has been explored extensively in post-processing respiratory rate calculations [16]. Therefore we assess EEMD as a strong baseline of comparison. EEMD was applied to the PPG signal to extract the IMFs using publicly available PyEMD library [27,28]. To reduce processing time and accommodate real-time constraints, we imposed a limitation of 5 iterations during the EMD process. Additionally, our data windows were restricted to 1 s to ensure real-time feasibility. As a result, we generated only 2 IMFs during the EMD. Based on visual inspection and comparison, we identified the second IMF, which exhibited the closest resemblance to the respiratory curve and contained the most relevant respiratory information, as the chosen IMF for further analysis and tracking.

Seq2Seq. After a series of preliminary experiments using simple feedforward, recurrent and convolutional architectures, we developed a hybrid model combining an autoencoder and a Seq2Seq model. An autoencoder (AE) is a type of unsupervised artificial neural network that aims to reconstruct its input at the output layer while imposing a condition on its hidden representations (e.g. size, distribution, sparsity). Autoencoders consist of an encoder that compresses the input data into a lower-dimensional representation, called the latent vector, while the decoder reconstructs the input from this latent representation. The use of autoencoders offers several advantages, such as dimensionality reduction, feature extraction, and new data generation. By compressing the input data into a lower-dimensional space, autoencoders can capture the most salient features and eliminate noise and redundant information [5,6].

Sequence-to-sequence is a type of supervised artificial neural network that aims to transform an input sequence to an output sequence. The Seq2Seq model also consists of an encoder and a decoder. The encoder processes the input sequence and converts it into a fixed-length latent representation [13,41].

In this study we used a Seq2Seq model in combination with an AE. Due to the different nature of the input and output sequences (ground-truth being a smooth signal and PPG containing fast oscillations), using only the Seq2Seq model resulted in high losses. To address this, an AE was introduced to extract the most important information or latent vector from the ground-truth signal. By generating a more sparse representation of the output signal, the AE helps to better match the characteristics of the PPG signal, making the overall model more effective in generating accurate results and reducing the losses encountered in the Seq2Seq approach. In this approach, the autoencoder accepts inductive respiratory chest strap signals as input and encodes the latent vector representation of the RIP signals. The latent representation becomes the ground truth for our Seq2Seq model, which utilizes the raw PPG to predict the encoded latent vector from the autoencoder to generate respiratory information from a PPG signal. The Seq2Seq structure then outputs a generated latent vector, which is passed as input to the previously trained decoder of our autoencoder to create generated respiratory signals.

Figure 3 represents the schematic of Seq2Seq model. The Seq2Seq component (Fig. 3A) starts with an input layer, followed by 2 consecutive Conv1D blocks. An add layer is applied to combine the outputs of two convolutional layers. This is followed by additional Conv1D layers with layer normalization and add layers

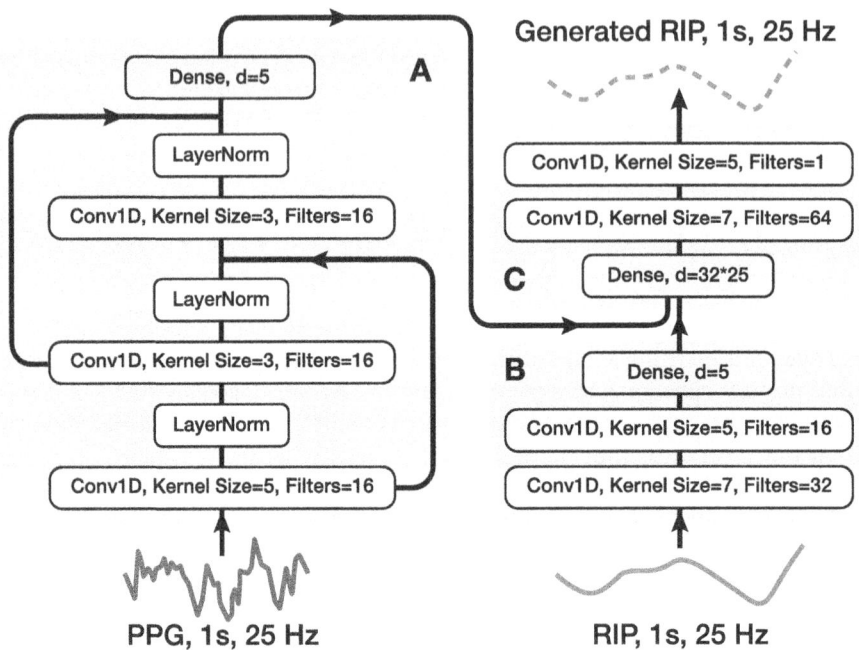

Fig. 3. The Seq2Seq model incorporates an autoencoder (AE) for RIP signals and an encoder for PPG, resulting in a hybrid model structure. A) PPG encoder: encodes raw PPG into latent representation of respiratory signals. B) RIP endoder: encodes RIP signals into latent representations for the decoder. This block was only used during training and was discarded at inference time C) RIP decoder: The generated latent representation of respiratory signals is given to the decoder to generate the respiratory signal. At inference time, the input signal to the decoder comes from the PPG encoder and the RIP encoder is discarded.

to further refine the representations. The output is then flattened and passed through a dense layer for final processing.

The autoencoder begins with an input layer, followed by a sequential layer. The encoder section (Fig. 3B) of the autoencoder includes Conv1D layers and a dense layer for dimensionality reduction. The encoder is followed by a sequential layer then the decoder (Fig. 3C) which is composed of dense layer and Conv1D layers for signal reconstruction. The whole model was developed using TensorFlow [1].

This approach enabled us to generate respiratory signals that closely resembled the original data. We utilized an Adam optimizer with a learning rate of 0.0001 and gradient clipping with a threshold of 0.5 to stabilize training. The mean squared error (MSE) loss function was employed to measure the discrepancy between the predicted respiratory signals and the ground truth. This helped ensure that the model was trained sufficiently without compromising its generalization capabilities.

GAN. A Generative Adversarial Network (GAN) is a type of machine learning model that consists of two main components: a generator and a discriminator. The generator aims to synthesize realistic samples, while the discriminator learns to distinguish between real and generated samples [14]. By training the generator to produce respiratory signals that closely resemble real signals, GANs offer a powerful tool for simulating realistic respiratory patterns. In this process, both parts of the GAN (generator and discriminator) are used during training. However, during the testing phase, the discriminator is no longer utilized for generating the output, resulting in significantly faster processing times. This efficiency allows the GAN-based model to generate accurate and realistic respiratory information in real-time applications. A Conditional GAN introduces additional conditioning information to both the generator and the discriminator, allowing for more targeted and controlled generation of samples [21].

A Conditional GAN will take pairs of real data samples and their conditions as well as pairs of fake or generated samples and intended conditions for training. Using feedback from the discriminator, the generator learns to produce data that is more realistic and aligns well with a given data pair condition. In our model, the positive pair (pertaining to ground truth samples) was defined as real PPG and RIP sensor signals. The negative pair (pertaining to generated samples) was defined as real PPG and generated RIP sensor signals.

In GANs, loss functions quantify the discrepancy between the generated samples and the real samples, providing a signal for the model to optimize its performance. Two commonly used loss functions in GANs are cross-entropy loss and Wasserstein loss. Cross-entropy loss measures the dissimilarity between the predicted distribution and the true distribution [46]. Wasserstein loss calculates the distance between the generated and real distributions using the Earth Mover's Distance. To stabilize training and encourage the generator to produce diverse samples, gradient penalty is utilized in conjunction with Wasserstein loss GANs. Gradient penalty introduces a regularization term that penalizes the discriminator for having large gradients, preventing it from overpowering the generator during training [15]. We employed Wasserstein loss, which proved to be effective in mitigating mode collapse and promoting diverse sample generation. We further incorporated gradient penalty to enhance generated signal quality. We used an RMSprop optimizer with a learning rate of 5e-5. The model was trained for 200 epochs.

In our model depicted in Fig. 4, the generator component (Fig. 4A) begins with an input layer, followed by a series of Conv1D layers. Each Conv1D layer is paired with a Leaky ReLU nonlinearity and LayerNorm. The discriminator component (Fig. 4B) also starts with an input layer, followed by multiple convolutional layers with a Leaky ReLU nonlinearity and LayerNorm layers. This model was developed using TensorFlow [1].

2.5 Respiratory Rate Estimation

To confirm the accuracy of the generated signal, an offline analysis of respiratory rate (RR) estimation on the 1 min test signal was performed. To accu-

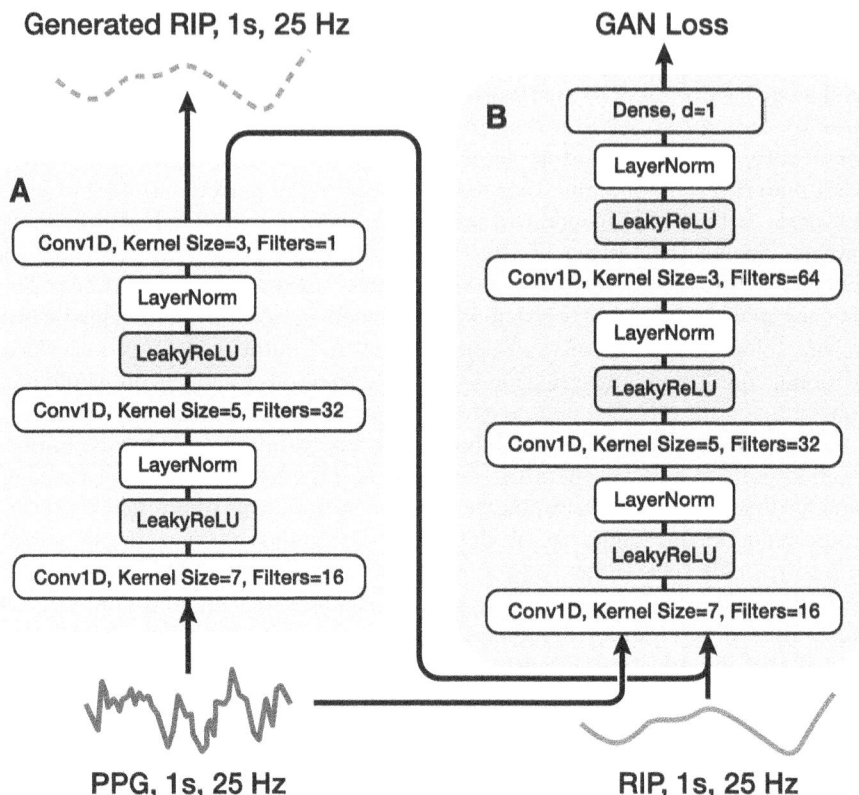

Fig. 4. Conditional GAN model showing a generator block and a discriminator block, A) The Generator tries to generate RIP signals based on the PPG conditioning input. B) the Discriminator computes the discriminator loss based on the input conditioning signal and the ground-truth RIP signal. If the input to the discriminator comes from a pair of ground truth RIP and its corresponding PPG, the block should detect the input as real; otherwise, if the generated RIP is paired with PPG, the discriminator should classify it as fake.

rately estimate RR from the real and generated signals obtained through our proposed system, we employed a custom peak detection pipeline. Firstly, we applied detrending to the signals, which helped improve the definition of peak occurrences, enhancing the accuracy of peak detection. Next, a moving average with a 1-s window was applied to the signals. This moving average served to smoothen the data and reduce any noise or fluctuations, providing a cleaner signal for further analysis. We then identify peak occurrences across the signals and store their indices to an array. To detect the valleys between the peaks, we determine the signal values between two consecutive peak indices and return the index of the minimum value. This algorithm effectively identified the peaks present in the signals, which corresponded to the peaks in the breathing cycles.

Once the peaks and valleys were identified, we proceeded to calculate the respiratory rate. This involved determining the number of peaks occurring within a given window range defined as peaks per minute. To achieve this, we counted the number of peaks within a specified window length of the signal and multiplied this rate by the sample rate to obtain the rate in peaks per second. Finally, we multiplied this value by 60 s to express the respiratory rate as peaks per minute. We calculated respiratory rate in windows of 30-s with a 29 s overlap. We defined the values to represent the breaths per-minute respiratory rate.

2.6 Breathing Depth

Breathing depth plays a significant role in differentiating between deep and shallow breathing. It serves as an indicator of the amount of inhaled air that fills the lungs during respiration [31]. To quantify breathing depths, we employed an amplitude measurement, which represents the difference between the peak and valley of each breath. For each subject, we calculated the breathing depth for every breath, obtaining individual depth scores. To compare the ground truth breathing depths with the generated breathing depths, we computed the average breathing depth scores for each subject. This allowed us to assess the accuracy and consistency of the generated respiratory signals in capturing the desired breathing depths.

Figure 5 demonstrates an example of breathing curve, highlighting the signal peaks and what is denoted as 1 breath and breathing depth.

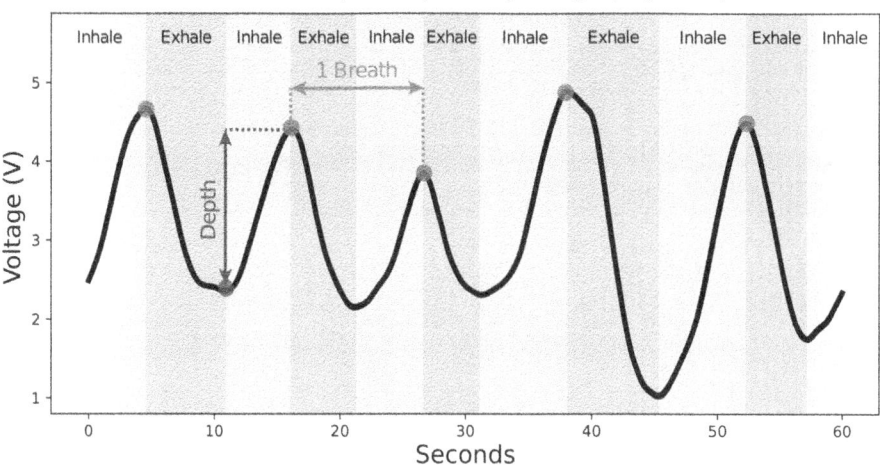

Fig. 5. Breathing curve characteristics: a 1-minute sample of the RIP signal is depicted with the peaks highlighted. Here RR, defined as the number of peaks in a minute, is five bpm. First, the distance between consecutive peaks and valleys is calculated for the depth score, and then this difference is averaged over the entire sequence.

2.7 Real-Time Implementation

The generated respiratory signal was streamed at a rate of 25 Hz. To enhance the accuracy of the signal and reduce high-frequency noise, we applied a 1 s window moving average. Smoothing the generated signal results in a more reliable representation of the respiratory pattern. Figure 6 illustrates an example of the streamed generated signal (in blue) along with the recorded PPG signal (in red). We then apply the aforementioned peak detection algorithm to identify respiratory rate as using a 20-s window length updated every 1 s. Next, we performed a weighted classification of the breathing phase based on the signal characteristics. By analyzing the slope of the signal, we classified it as either breathing in or breathing out. A positive slope indicated the onset of inhalation, while a negative slope indicated the onset of exhalation. The duration of the positive or negative slope influenced the weighting or confidence assigned to each breathing phase classification. A longer duration of a particular slope resulted in a higher weighted classification, indicating a higher level of confidence in the assigned phase. Breathing phase was detected every 1 s and stored in a phase classification array.

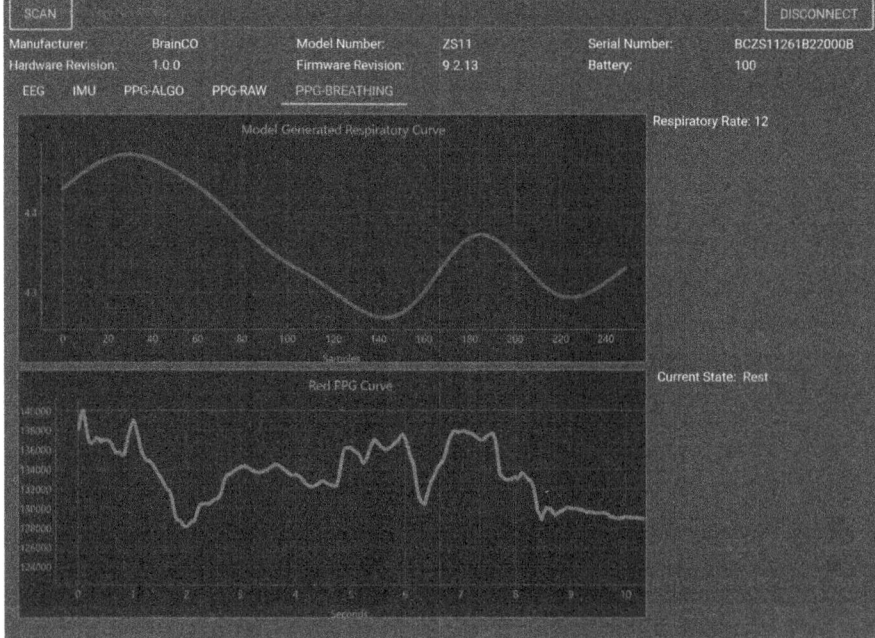

Fig. 6. GUI: In the study focusing on the breathing generation based on PPG, the PPG- BREATHING tab of the developed SDK is used. Other tabs won't be discussed as they are out of the scope of this paper. In this tab, the model-generated respiratory curve is displayed at top and Red PPG curve at the bottom. Respiratory Rate estimated based on our generated signal is shown beside the top plot. (Color figure online)

To identify a complete breath, we analyzed the stream of breathing state classifiers. By monitoring the transitions between breathing in and breathing out states, we determined the occurrence of a complete breath. This sliding 20-s window (with an overlap of 19-s) allowed for a dynamic classification of breathing phase.

3 Results

In this study, we utilized three different methods to track the breathing cycle. Figure 7 shows an example of the breathing signals generated by these methods (Fig. 7C), along with PPG (Fig. 7A) and the ground truth signal (Fig. 7B) recorded from a RIP sensor. The models produced real-time signals every second, resulting in 60 windows that were then concatenated, smoothed and detrended. Since PPG and RIP have different ranges, for visualization all generated signals were min-max normalized.

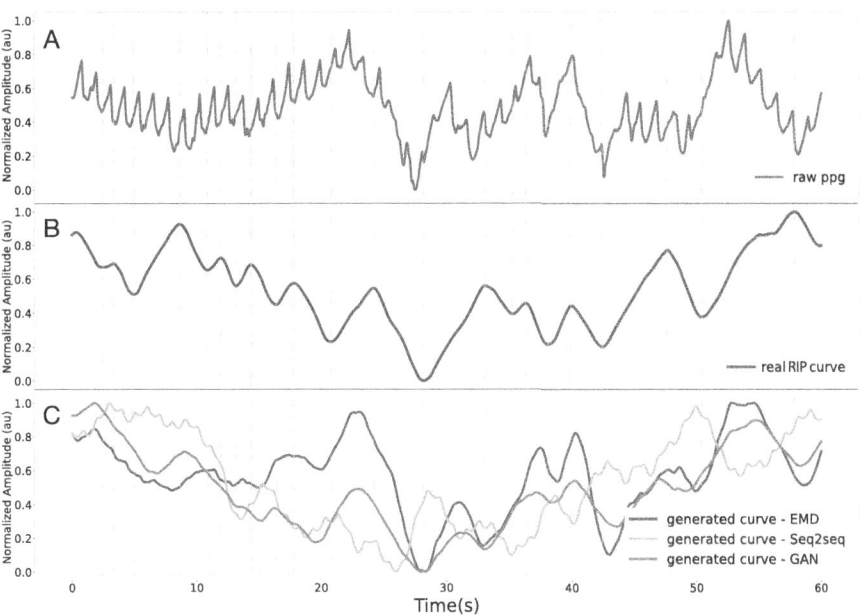

Fig. 7. Model performance comparison: A) A sample of PPG signal given as the input to the models, B) The ground-truth signal with vertical dashed lines highlighting the start and end of each breathing phase (inhale or exhale). C) Generated signals by the three models for the given PPG signal. The GAN-generated signal is more accurately following the ground-truth.

It is important to note that the generated signals have a 1-s delay compared to the real signal. The example in the figure was intentionally selected to demonstrate the strengths and limitations of our proposed method. Since the EMD method does not rely on supervised learning, its output resembles the PPG signal more than the desired RIP signal. As shown in the figure, the GAN-generated signal closely follows the ground truth compared to the other two methods. However, the GAN algorithm faces challenges in tracking very shallow breaths (<0.01 au) and fast breaths with higher frequencies (>20 bpm). Since any breathing period with a bpm above 20 is defined as non-normal breathing, rapid breathing, or tachypnea [26] we define this algorithm as qualified for the normal breathing range.

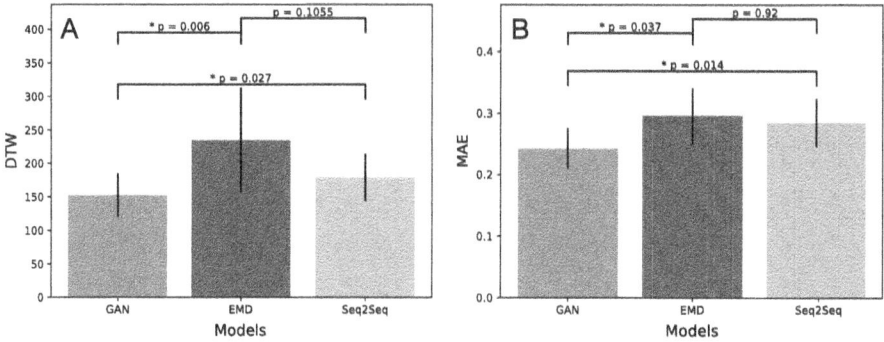

Fig. 8. Quantitative comparison of models: A) As one measure of dissimilarity between generated signal and ground-truth signal, average DTW distances over 1-minute test signal for all subjects were compared for all three methods, GAN method shows better performance with statistical significance. B) All three method's MAE between generated and ground-truth signals were also compared to reflect the error between the two. Similarly GAN-generated signal with less error showed closer behavior to ground-truth with statistical significance.

To quantitatively assess the performance of three methods in tracking the ground-truth breathing cycle, Dynamic Time Warping (DTW) and Mean Absolute Error (MAE) were utilized. DTW is a technique employed to measure the similarity between two time series sequences of different lengths. In comparison to cross-correlation, DTW excels in local pattern matching, enabling it to focus on identifying similar segments of the signals. This effectiveness becomes evident in scenarios where certain segments hold greater importance than others [33]. Specifically, in our generated data, where the signal closely resembles the ground-truth during specific segments of normal breathing, DTW distance served as one of the measures to evaluate the performance of the methods quantitatively. Generated respiratory signals using each method were compared with ground-truth over the 60s test data. As a second measure, the normalized generated signals were compared to the ground truth using MAE. MAE is a metric that calculates the average absolute difference between the generated signals and the ground truth, providing a quantitative measure of the overall accuracy of the generated signals in relation to the ground truth. In order to compare the statistical difference, the results were then tested for normality using the Shapiro-Wilk test showing non-normal behavior in some distributions. To simultaneously compare the performance of the three methods, a Friedman rank test is utilized, followed by a post hoc pairwise test employing the Wilcoxon signed-rank test. Lastly, Holm's method is used to adjust the significance thresholds (alpha). All statistical analysis were performed using SciPy [44] and statsmodels [35] libraries. The results of DTW and MAE analysis are shown in Fig. 8 for test data. Both measures reveal that the GAN performance surpasses the other two methods with statistical significance.

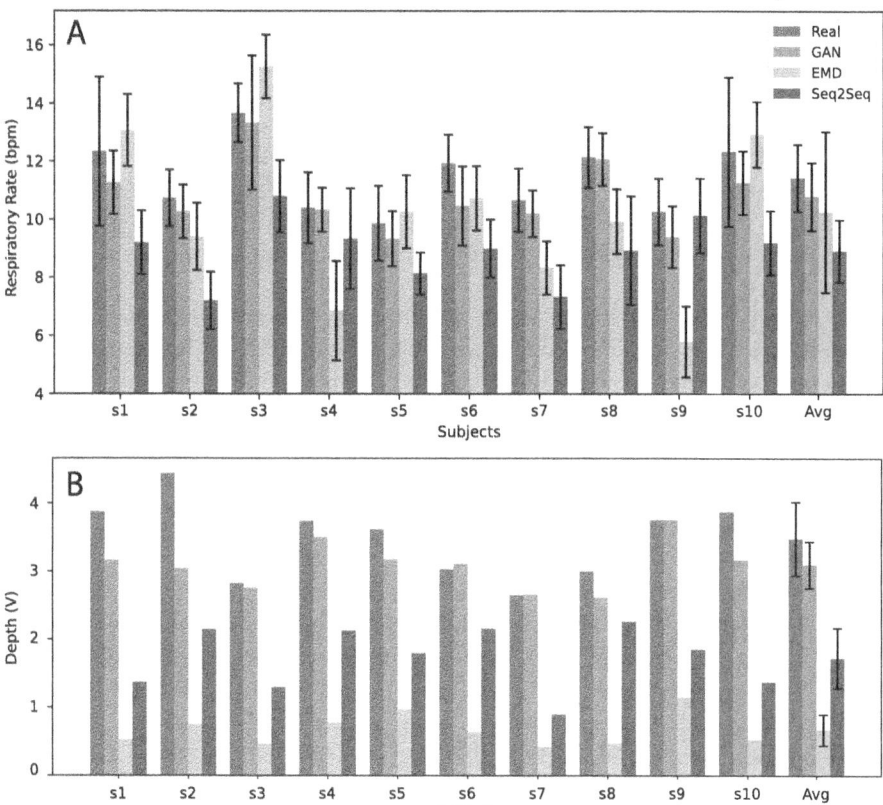

Fig. 9. Breathing measures: A) Average RR estimation over 1 min test signal, based on the generated signals by three models are compared with RR of ground-truth for all subjects individually as well as average over all subjects. B) Depth scores for generated signals and the ground-truth curve are compared for all individual subjects and average of all subjects. These graphs shows the superior performance of GAN-generated signal in monitoring breathing pattern.

After generating the breathing curves, we proceeded to estimate the RR for each subject using all methods. In Fig. 9A, we compared the average RR estimation over a 30-s sliding window of the generated test signals with the ground-truth signal for each subject. Furthermore, we calculated the MAE between repetitions for each subject. This metric provides an assessment of the consistency and accuracy of the RR estimates across different repetitions. The average MAE overall subjects for GAN, EMD and Seq2Seq is 1.47, 2.28 and 2.83 bpm respectively. The MAE values provide insights into the overall variability and precision of the RR estimations, contributing to the assessment of the reliability of the GAN-generated signals in tracking and estimating respiratory rate. The results demonstrate minimal differences between the GAN-generated and ground-truth signal, indicating a high level of similarity in the RR estimations. Alongside the estimation of respiratory rate, we also computed the average breathing depth during the one-minute test data for each subject. Figure 9B displays the corresponding results for each subject, comparing the values obtained from the real RIP signal with those generated by our algorithm. These results underscore the capability of the GAN generated signals to closely track and mimic the actual breathing depth. The two other methods show inconsistent behaviour considering different features. EMD is closer to real signal in RR estimation compared with Seq2Seq, while Seq2Seq is better in estimating breath depths compared with EMD.

To evaluate the real-time usage of our method, we recorded demos from two subjects, one male and one female, while they were actively breathing. These demos provide valuable insights into how our method performs in real-time scenarios and can be used to showcase its potential applications and benefits. The demo video is available at this hyperlink.

4 Discussion

Real-time monitoring of breathing is of significant importance, particularly in outpatient settings where low-cost wearables that are comfortable and easy to wear are essential. In this study, we developed an algorithm utilizing a low-frequency PPG sensor, enabling real-time assessment of breathing with a 1-s latency.

Our results demonstrate the feasibility of utilizing a low-frequency PPG for monitoring breathing. The algorithm's performance was evaluated on 10 subjects, revealing the GAN's ability to generate a reliable tracking of the real respiratory signal despite the low sampling rate of the PPG (25 Hz), which resulted in a low number of samples per window (25 samples). Importantly, the GAN outperformed the other two methods, namely EMD and Seq2Seq. This is attributed to the specific challenge of the low-frequency nature of the PPG signal (25 Hz). While EMD and Seq2Seq focused on capturing the low-frequency oscillations present in the PPG, only the GAN was capable of effectively tracking the relatively higher frequency content present in the ground-truth signal. The dissimilarity between the three methods and the ground-truth signal was quantified using DTW and MAE, acknowledging that some level of variation is expected due to the different sources of the signals (RIP vs. PPG). Although the magnitude of the DTW distance itself does not determine the method's goodness, it is evident from Fig. 8A that the GAN exhibits less dissimilarity and statistically significant differences compared to the other methods. Figure 8B further supports these observations by comparing the performance of the three methods using MAE. Figure 9A illustrates the close resemblance of the GAN-based RR estimations to the ground truth, with an average mean absolute error (MAE) of 1.47 bpm. Additionally, Fig. 9B demonstrates the accuracy of the GAN-generated signals in estimating breathing depth (Table 1).

Table 1. Comparison of our method and Selvakumar [36]

Paper	RR MAE	Sampling Rate	Window Size
Karman et al.	1.47 bpm	25 Hz	1 s
Selvakumar et al.	1 bpm	125 Hz	5 s

In the recent literature, there is a scarcity of studies using low-frequency PPG for real-time breathing monitoring. In comparison to Selvakumar [36], their method achieved MAE less than 1 bpm over various breathing frequency ranges. However, it should be noted that their approach employed a PPG with a higher sampling rate of 125 Hz and relied on 5 s of data (625 samples per window), whereas our algorithm achieves comparable accuracy with only 1 s of data using a 25 Hz PPG sensor (25 samples per window). Overall, our results align with the latest research in the field and are applicable to any PPG-based system, given the 25 Hz sampling rate.

One of the limitations of our method is that it may encounter challenges in generating the respiratory signal accurately when the subject exhibits fast and shallow breathing, as can occur during talking or abnormal breathing patterns. One possible approach to addressing this limitation would involve utilizing a higher sampling rate for the PPG data. With a higher sampling rate, our method may have better captured the nuances of fast and shallow breathing patterns, thereby potentially improving the generation of the respiratory signal in such scenarios. Additionally, conducting a real-time evaluation study would allow us to assess the algorithm's performance in real-world scenarios. Moreover, it is important to investigate the user experience and ease of use for operators. This setup and real-time algorithm will be employed in a clinical study conducted in a hospital to aid children with pain control after surgery, with the aim of reducing the use of opioids.

In this study, we explored different signal processing and machine learning algorithms, such as EMD, Seq2Seq, and GAN, to track the breathing process in real-time using a low-power PPG signal mounted on a headband. Our developed GAN algorithm showed promising results in accurately tracking the breathing cycle. Our findings demonstrate the effectiveness of our algorithm for real-time and low-latency breathing monitoring using low-frequency PPG, highlighting its potential applications in pain control and mindful breathing practices. PPG sensors integrated into wearable devices, such as smartwatches, provide a convenient and continuous means for real-time breathing monitoring. Leveraging this technology presents an opportunity to track the breathing cycle in diverse situations, prompting the need for user-friendly solutions. While inductive chest strap sensors are commonly used in hospital settings, their discomfort limits their widespread adoption. Our proposed tool addresses these limitations by offering an easy-to-deploy, comfortable, and user-friendly wearable device for real-time breathing monitoring. It provides an effective and accessible solution for at-home respiratory monitoring with potential applications in various healthcare domains. This sets the stage for future research conducting online evaluation studies to further validate and improve our method.

Acknowledgments. We want to acknowledge Ken Glass at Dell Technologies for providing state-of-the-art machine learning work stations.
We acknowledge Plux Biosignals for providing our data acquisition toolkit.
We also want to thank Lawrence Franchini for pushing us to tackle respiratory sensing as well as the BrainCo team members who were able to participate in our data collection procedures.

References

1. Abadi, M., et al.: TensorFlow: large-scale machine learning on heterogeneous systems (2015). https://www.tensorflow.org/
2. Alian, A.A., Shelley, K.H.: Photoplethysmography. Best Pract. Res. Clin. Anaesthesiol. **28**, 395–406 (2014). https://doi.org/10.1016/j.bpa.2014.08.006
3. Alian, A.A., Shelley, K.H.: PPG in clinical monitoring. In: Photoplethysmography, pp. 341–359. Elsevier (2022)
4. Azmal, G.M., Al-Jumaily, A., Al-Jaafreh, M.: Continuous measurement of oxygen saturation level using photoplethysmography signal (2006). https://doi.org/10.1109/ICBPE.2006.348646
5. Baldi, P.: Autoencoders, unsupervised learning, and deep architectures. In: ICML Unsupervised and Transfer Learning (2012). https://doi.org/10.1561/2200000006
6. Barot, V., Patel, D.R.: A physiological signal compression approach using optimized spindle convolutional auto-encoder in mhealth applications. Biomed. Signal Process. Control **73**, 103436 (2022). https://doi.org/10.1016/j.bspc.2021.103436
7. Boccignone, G., D'Amelio, A., Ghezzi, O., Grossi, G., Lanzarotti, R.: An evaluation of non-contact photoplethysmography-based methods for remote respiratory rate estimation. Sensors **23**, 3387 (2023). https://doi.org/10.3390/s23073387
8. BrainCo. https://brainco.tech/. Accessed 24 July 2023
9. Chen, L., Liu, X., Peng, L., Wu, M.: Deep learning based multimodal complex human activity recognition using wearable devices. Appl. Intell. **51** (2021). https://doi.org/10.1007/s10489-020-02005-7
10. Drigas, A., Mitsea, E.: Breathing: a powerfull tool for physical & neuropsychological regulation. the role of mobile apps. Technium Soc. Sci. J. **28**, 135 (2022)
11. Faust-Christmann, C.A., Taetz, B., Zolynski, G., Zimmermann, T., Bleser, G.: A biofeedback app to instruct abdominal breathing (breathing-mentor): pilot experiment. JMIR Mhealth Uhealth **7**(9), e13703 (2019)

12. FocusCalm. https://focuscalm.com/. Accessed 24 July 2023
13. Gehring, J., Auli, M., Grangier, D., Yarats, D., Dauphin, Y.N.: Convolutional sequence to sequence learning (2017)
14. Goodfellow, I.J., et al.: Generative adversarial networks (2014)
15. Gulrajani, I., Ahmed, F., Arjovsky, M., Dumoulin, V., Courville, A.: Improved training of Wasserstein GANs (2017)
16. Hadiyoso, S., Dewi, E.M., Wijayanto, I.: Comparison of EMD, VMD and EEMD methods in respiration wave extraction based on PPG waves. J. Phys. Conf. Ser. **1577**, 012040 (2020). https://doi.org/10.1088/1742-6596/1577/1/012040
17. Karlen, W., Raman, S., Ansermino, J.M., Dumont, G.A.: Multiparameter respiratory rate estimation from the photoplethysmogram. IEEE Trans. Biomed. Eng. **60**, 1946–1953 (2013). https://doi.org/10.1109/TBME.2013.2246160
18. Khalid, S.G., Zhang, J., Chen, F., Zheng, D.: Blood pressure estimation using photoplethysmography only: comparison between different machine learning approaches. J. Healthc. Eng. **2018**, 1–13 (2018). https://doi.org/10.1155/2018/1548647
19. Khamis, A., Kusy, B., Chou, C.T., Hu, W.: Wirelax: towards real-time respiratory biofeedback during meditation using wifi. Ad Hoc Netw. **107**, 102226 (2020). https://doi.org/10.1016/j.adhoc.2020.102226
20. Lukic, Y.X., Teepe, G.W., Fleisch, E., Kowatsch, T.: Breathing as an input modality in a gameful breathing training app (breeze 2): development and evaluation study. JMIR Serious Games **10**, e39186 (2022). https://doi.org/10.2196/39186
21. Mirza, M., Osindero, S.: Conditional generative adversarial nets (2014)
22. Mohan, P.M., Nisha, A.A., Nagarajan, V., Jothi, E.S.J.: Measurement of arterial oxygen saturation (spo<inf>2</inf>) using PPG optical sensor, pp. 1136–1140. IEEE (2016). https://doi.org/10.1109/ICCSP.2016.7754330
23. Motin, M.A., Karmakar, C.K., Palaniswami, M.: Ensemble empirical mode decomposition with principal component analysis: a novel approach for extracting respiratory rate and heart rate from photoplethysmographic signal. IEEE J. Biomed. Health Inform. **22**, 766–774 (2018). https://doi.org/10.1109/JBHI.2017.2679108
24. Nicolò, A., Massaroni, C., Schena, E., Sacchetti, M.: The importance of respiratory rate monitoring: from healthcare to sport and exercise. Sensors **20**(21), 6396 (2020)
25. Park, C., Lee, B.: Real-time estimation of respiratory rate from a photoplethysmogram using an adaptive lattice notch filter. BioMedical Engi. OnLine **13**, 170 (2014). https://doi.org/10.1186/1475-925X-13-170
26. Park, S.B., Khattar, D.: Tachypnea (2023)
27. Pele, O., Werman, M.: A linear time histogram metric for improved SIFT matching. In: Forsyth, D., Torr, P., Zisserman, A. (eds.) ECCV 2008. LNCS, vol. 5304, pp. 495–508. Springer, Heidelberg (2008). https://doi.org/10.1007/978-3-540-88690-7_37
28. Pele, O., Werman, M.: Fast and robust earth mover's distances. In: 2009 IEEE 12th International Conference on Computer Vision, pp. 460–467. IEEE (2009)
29. Plux. https://www.pluxbiosignals.com/products/inductive-respiration-rip-sensor. Accessed 24 July 2023
30. Prana.co. https://prana.co/. Accessed 24 July 2023
31. Rahman, M.M., et al.: Breathebuddy: tracking real-time breathing exercises for automated biofeedback using commodity earbuds. Proc. ACM Hum.-Comput. Interact. **6**, 1–18 (2022). https://doi.org/10.1145/3546748
32. Ribeiro, H.D.M., et al.: ECG-based real-time arrhythmia monitoring using quantized deep neural networks: a feasibility study. Comput. Biol. Med. **143**, 105249 (2022)

33. Sakoe, H., Chiba, S.: Dynamic programming algorithm optimization for spoken word recognition. IEEE Trans. Acoust. Speech Signal Process. **26** (1978). https://doi.org/10.1109/TASSP.1978.1163055
34. Sangeeta, B., Laxmi, S.: A real time analysis of PPG signal for measurement of SPO2 and pulse rate. Int. J. Comput. Appl. **36**, 45–50 (2011)
35. Seabold, S., Perktold, J.: Statsmodels: econometric and statistical modeling with python. In: 9th Python in Science Conference (2010)
36. Selvakumar, K., et al.: Realtime PPG based respiration rate estimation for remote health monitoring applications. Biomed. Signal Process. Control **77**, 103746 (2022). https://doi.org/10.1016/j.bspc.2022.103746
37. Sharma, H.: Extraction of respiratory rate from PPG using ensemble empirical mode decomposition with kalman filter. Electron. Lett. **56**, 650–653 (2020). https://doi.org/10.1049/el.2020.0566
38. Shih, C.H.I., Tomita, N., Lukic, Y.X., Reguera, Á.H., Fleisch, E., Kowatsch, T.: Breeze: smartphone-based acoustic real-time detection ofbreathing phases for a gamified biofeedback breathing training. Proc. ACM Interact. Mob. Wearable Ubiquitous Technol. **3**, 1–30 (2019). https://doi.org/10.1145/3369835
39. Shuzan, M.N.I., et al.: Machine learning-based respiration rate and blood oxygen saturation estimation using photoplethysmogram signals. Bioengineering **10**, 167 (2023). https://doi.org/10.3390/bioengineering10020167
40. Soroushmojdehi, R., Javadzadeh, S., Pedrocchi, A., Gandolla, M.: Transfer learning in hand movement intention detection based on surface electromyography signals. Front. Neurosci. **16** (2022). https://doi.org/10.3389/fnins.2022.977328
41. Sutskever, I., Vinyals, O., Le, Q.V.: Sequence to sequence learning with neural networks (2014)
42. Tanaka, M., Kakuma, T., Asada, T.: Utility of paced breathing tablet guidance apparatus with real-time feedback on autonomic function for individuals with mild cognitive impairment: a pilot study. Psychogeriatrics **23**, 434–441 (2023). https://doi.org/10.1111/psyg.12950
43. Ullah, I., Hussain, M., ul Haq Qazi, E., Aboalsamh, H.: An automated system for epilepsy detection using EEG brain signals based on deep learning approach. Expert Syst. Appl. **107**, 61–71 (2018). https://doi.org/10.1016/j.eswa.2018.04.021
44. Virtanen, P., et al.: SciPy 1.0: fundamental algorithms for scientific computing in python. Nat. Methods **17**, 261–272 (2020). https://doi.org/10.1038/s41592-019-0686-2
45. Wu, Z., Huang, N.E.: Ensemble empirical mode decomposition: a noise-assisted data analysis method. Adv. Adapt. Data Anal. **01**, 1–41 (2009). https://doi.org/10.1142/S1793536909000047
46. Xu, J., Ren, X., Lin, J., Sun, X.: Diversity-promoting GAN: a cross-entropy based generative adversarial network for diversified text generation, pp. 3940–3949. Association for Computational Linguistics (2018). https://doi.org/10.18653/v1/D18-1428

Navigating Health Applications Realms: Consent Challenges and User Empowerment in European Law

Petra Müllerová(✉)

Lund University, Box 188, 221 00 Lund, Sweden
petra.mullerova@jur.lu.se

Abstract. This study delves into the landscape of health applications within online markets. These applications, offering health-related functionalities, have become integral to the lives of European citizens. The transformation of healthcare delivery, accelerated by the pace of modern life and accentuated by the COVID-19 pandemic, has elevated health applications from conveniences to essential tools capable of optimising diagnoses, self-awareness, and doctor-patient collaborations. As European societies undergo demographic shifts, with an ageing population, the significance of health applications grows. The elderly population has implications for healthcare demand as longer lifespans necessitate sustained medical interventions. These technologies, though often perceived as youth-oriented, offer substantial benefits for older individuals, a significant portion of whom grapple with chronic ailments, particularly in rural areas with limited access. The article highlights the challenge of obtaining valid user consent for health data processing, which is a cornerstone of health data protection. Issues such as granularity of consent, transparency, and power imbalances are explored in the context of health applications. The study emphasises the need for informed, unambiguous, and freely given consent, noting the discrepancies between legal requirements and actual practices. Concluding, the research suggests that despite existing legal safeguards, there are gaps in implementing robust data protection practices in health applications. The study proposes empowering users with knowledge about their rights and encouraging best practices among application manufacturers to bridge the divide between legal provisions and actual data protection. This approach aims to ensure the integrity and security of users' health data in the realm of health applications.

Keywords: Health applications · Protection of personal health data · GDPR

1 Introduction

Online markets on our smartphones, such as Google Play and the App Store, suggest up to 370,000 health applications daily. Remarkably, these digital health companions have ingrained themselves in the lives of European citizens, with adoption rates ranging from 22% to 44%, contingent upon the geographic context [1]. The metamorphosis of healthcare delivery, driven by the accelerating pace of life and accentuated by the transformative impact of the COVID-19 pandemic, has elevated the stature of health applications from novel conveniences to indispensable tools. Their potential extends beyond mere patient empowerment to encompass optimised diagnoses, heightened self-awareness, and fortified doctor-patient collaborations [2]. Beyond the individual realm, the burgeoning landscape of health applications holds promise for healthcare systems, offering prospects of substantial financial savings [2].

As the demographic fabric of European societies evolves, marked by a diminishing working-age population juxtaposed against an ageing citizenry, the significance of health applications amplifies. The surge in the elderly population, particularly those aged over 85, has profound implications for healthcare demands, as longer life expectancies necessitate augmented and sustained medical interventions [3]. Paradoxically, while these technologies are often perceived as the domain of the young [15], they have the potential to yield outsized benefits for older individuals, more than 55% of whom grapple with chronic ailments and rely on consistent medical care [4]. Moreover, this demographic shift assumes particular importance in the context of rural areas, where access to traditional healthcare often entails arduous journeys to urban centres [3]. Health applications, underpinned by the virtual realm, mitigate this geographical barrier, bridging the gap and offering a modality of healthcare delivery aligned with contemporary sensibilities. Today's generation of older people (over 60 years old) represents the first generation that could master modern technologies to a greater extent for the benefit of their health. In 2020, more than 90% of this group in Sweden stated that they regularly work with the Internet. The situation is different in each Member state; however, the average is 60% of older people with regular internet access.

In the European Union (EU) legal framework, the trend toward regulating health applications began with the 2014 European Commission (Commission) Green Paper on mobile health [5]. It described health applications as the future of European healthcare and promoted the 'qualified self' principle to achieve sustainable healthcare for the EU population. This principle consists of measuring specific life parameters to keep oneself in good condition based on the advice of health applications without the healthcare professional's supervision.

If health applications are to be the future of our healthcare system, it is not enough to simply support development and motivate citizens to use them. These advances have implications for digital privacy and may increase the risk of inadvertent breaches of client confidentiality [14]. Individual privacy is a fundamental human right and must be protected [29]. The Charter of Fundamental Rights of the European Union, in addition to the general protection of privacy, also regulates personal data and guarantees everyone the right to protect their personal data [31]. Member states and the EU as a whole must also ensure the safety of health applications. According to a BBC study of 5,000 health apps, more than 80% do not meet the standards set by UK legislation [6]. The shortcomings stem not only from the failure to meet the standards from the creation phase but also from a lack of regular updates in the scientific and security fields. And out of 83% of health applications, only 1% of all downloaded health apps make up [7]. Based on the ORCHA report from 2022, users' two severe concerns about using health apps have been identified in particular: i) protection of personal data and their privacy, ii) scientifically based treatment [8]. Both users and healthcare providers share the most significant concern, which revolves around whether the health applications provide scientific, evidence-based treatment [20]. Almost half of the users expressed concern that AI in the form of a chatbot in a health application cannot provide them with scientifically based treatment that is equivalent to the treatment provided by a doctor. Both areas are regulated by European law, specifically by the General Data Protection Regulation 2016/679 (GDPR) [33] and Regulation on Medical Devices 2017/745 [35]. Suppose a health application is considered a medical device. In that case, the standards for security, scientific evidence and data protection are higher than for other products (including health applications not certified as medical devices). Most health applications meet the requirements for being considered medical devices [16]. However, over 80% are not registered as medical devices [10]. This is caused by the Court of Justice of the European Union (CJEU) decision that the device shall be seen as medical only if intended for a medical purpose [11]. Health applications mainly declare themselves not to be intended for medical purposes but for the welfare of users. For this reason, it may not meet the stricter safety rules to protect the user's health. It is impossible for health applications to not comply with the rules for protecting personal data established by the GDPR. However, does this arrangement provide sufficient protection for users of health applications who do not always have advanced abilities to navigate new technologies? One in ten people do not use e-services for fear that their personal data will be accessed by others, and one in seven for fear of hackers getting access [9]. In this article, I will focus on researching legal provisions that protect personal data, especially health data, of the users of health applications. The study aims to answer whether the users' data of these applications is sufficiently protected or their data is at risk.

2 The Protection of Health Data in Health Applications

Personal health data has always been considered one of the most sensitive. Not only because they often reveal our weaknesses, disorders, predispositions, or habits. But also, genetic predispositions can affect our offspring, preventing us from pursuing a career in certain areas or disadvantage our societal position. For this reason, ethical and legislative protections generally require medical professionals to keep patients' medical records confidential unless the patient allows them to disclose it. Therefore, it is not a surprise that 35% of people are concerned about the security of their personal data that they entrust to health applications [10].

A recent American study conducted on three thousand patients revealed that despite the medical secret, 58% of patients can still not trust their GP [12]. Their most common concerns are embarrassment, fear of judgment, and avoiding lectures. Patients are most likely to lie about their mental health, frequency of exercise, and alcohol consumption. They also often lie about other topics, including diet, drug use, sexual activity, and smoking [22]. People don't lie about this data only to medical professionals but to all of society. In the area of sensitive information such as sex life or bad habits (smoking, alcohol consumption), people do not want to share this data with anyone. They fear this data might harm them in their private lives. Unfortunately, this research did not focus on health applications. Therefore, on the one hand, it can be assumed that people will not tend to tell the truth about health applications either. On the other hand, young people between 18 and 24 confirmed in the ORCHA survey that they also use health applications because they find them trustworthy and avoid contact with a health professional who could judge them for their bad habits [8]. The results are controversial because the 2022 study suggests that younger people, in particular, may be less likely to use technology for mental health, and they report a low preference for online mental health care compared to face-to-face treatment [13]. However, the truth of the health data entered into the application does not change the fact that all this data must be protected. Due to the complexity of the GDPR, in the following text, I will focus only on processing health data, as it must take place within the framework of every health application.

Based on the perception of this data as highly sensitive, the health data in health applications belongs to the category of special data already mentioned by the Oviedo Convention [30] and later regulated in the framework of the Data Protection Directive [37] and later amended as part of the GDPR. Since the GDPR is a regulation and not a directive, it is directly applicable and does not require transposition into national law. Even so, it has been transposed by most Member states, given that some articles allow for adopting certain national exceptions. The GDPR guarantees harmonised regulation, which is essential in this area for users, authorities and especially companies processing personal health data. It is, therefore, possible to market a health application that is subject to uniform criteria within all Member states. This requirement was essential for sensitive data such as health data. First, the meaning of 'health data' needs to be interpreted. In the framework of European law, the definition in Article 4, paragraph 15 GDPR is used: 'means personal data related to the physical or mental health of a natural person, including the provision of health care services, which reveal information about his or her health status.'

Since health data is taken in the context of that definition in a broader sense, health data is not limited to health care. Thus, health data also include parameters measured or observed, whether by the individual himself (the most common use of health applications), by the person caring for this individual or by a device used by the individual. In this strict sense, it is, therefore, possible to consider health data, for example, a menu compiled by a trainer at the gym, data recorded in a calorie counting application, and blood pressure measured by a home blood pressure monitor. A broader sense of health data thus makes it possible to protect the data of individuals even in situations where they are not aware that it is sensitive data.

GDPR defines the term 'processing of personal data' as an action or set of actions that may or may not be carried out based on an automated process. The regulation provides us with an open list of actions that can be taken to process personal data, which consists of collection, recording, organisation, structuring, storage, adaptation or alteration, retrieval, consultation, use, disclosure by transmission, dissemination, or otherwise making available, alignment or combination, restriction, erasure or destruction. The legislators have considered the possibility of further development of the use of personal data and, for this reason, have left the enumeration open to include new processes within this definition. In this sense, I have to constate that, in general, the majority of health applications are processing the users' health data. They mainly collect, store, record and use them for the user, themselves or third parties. The processing of health data is addressed in Article 9, paragraph 1 of the GDPR, which specifies that the processing of health data (as well as all other data within a special category) should be prohibited to protect the data subject. Therefore, these data are so strictly protected that they should not be processed. So how can some authorities encounter processing health data in the framework of public health care, for example, through the patient's medical record? Does it mean that all manufacturers of health applications are illegally processing health data? Despite this strict prohibition to process any health data, GDPR formulates a general exception in Recital 52:

Derogating from the prohibition on processing special categories of personal data should also be allowed when provided for in Union or Member State law and subject to suitable safeguards, so as to protect personal data and other fundamental rights [...]

The Recital specifies that processing is possible exclusively in the case of a sufficient guarantee of personal data protection, regardless of whether the guarantee is at the national or European level. Is the provision of this criterion adequate protection for health data? The legislators did not leave the exemption provision only in the recital framework, given that the regulation's preamble is presented as an explanatory statement. For clear bindingness, exceptions to the processing of this data category are defined in Article 9(2). The paragraph contains ten exceptions which, as required by recital 53, are granted exclusively for health-related purposes only where necessary to achieve those purposes for the benefit of natural persons and society. It should be added that this exception does not apply only to the public sector but to all processors of health data, including manufacturers of health applications. The exceptions can be divided into two groups: those created in the interest of an individual and those made in the public interest, i.e., in the interest of the whole society. The specific position between these two groups represents the exception cited in paragraph 2, letter (e), which allows the processing of the subject's data in case the data subject has already disclosed them. The subject's data can be used there to benefit the natural person and the companies. A presumption is created that if the data subjects have voluntarily disclosed the data, they have effectively consented to its use by others. This action does not alter the subject's rights to correct or delete the data.

In the context of the interests of the natural person, this includes letter a) consent given by the natural person for a specific purpose and letter c) where processing is necessary to protect the vital interests of the data subject or another natural person. The natural person's consent conditions will be discussed in detail in the chapter below because consent represents the most common measure used by manufacturers of health applications. The applicability of letter c) predicates the fulfilment of several non-cumulative conditions, namely that the data subject is not physically or legally capable of giving consent. This exception is mainly used in circumstances where it is necessary to save a life or prevent harm, and the data subject is unable to give consent, either because of their physical, mental, or legal capacity. It is assumed that this situation can occur within health applications, especially if it is a monitoring application. In this case, the application manufacturer has the right to share all life-saving data with medical professionals. This situation will probably be unique, and it is not certain that this data will be delivered on time to the people needing it. Hypothetically, however, this exception can also be used in the case of health applications.

To introduce the second group of exceptions aimed at the public benefit, i.e., the benefit of society, it is necessary to return to the purpose defined in Recital 53 and clarify the main concept. If Recital specifies the processing of health data for health-related purposes benefiting the whole society, it means processing data to protect public health. The term 'public health' is defined in the framework of Regulation 1338/2008 as follows:

shall mean all elements related to health, namely health status, including morbidity and disability, the determinants having an effect on that health status, health care needs, resources allocated to health care, the provision of, and universal access to, health care as well as health care expenditure and financing, and the causes of mortality. [34]

Surprisingly, despite Recital 53 explicitly mentioning health-related purposes as the object of exceptions in the public interest, only two exceptions defined in paragraph 2, namely letters (h) and (i), fall within the scope of the appeal of protecting public health. The first exception deals with the issue of preventive and occupational medicine. Information processing primarily protects employees or the general population or adjusts the provision of health, social care or treatment, or health systems and services management. The second exception even mentions that data processing, in this case, is for reasons of public interest to protect public health. It is about preventing or combating health threats, such as protecting against serious cross-border threats to health or ensuring high standards of quality and safety of health care and medicinal products or medical devices. These provisions apply to health applications only in the event that a public authority requests this data in the public interest. Again, it is hypothetically possible that the manufacturer will release data under these circumstances, but the probability that such data will be required is very low.

Although the other exceptions do not specifically refer to the public interest in public health, they all pursue other public interests vital to society. Letter (d) governs the operation of any foundation, association or other not-for-profit body with a political, philosophical, religious or trade union interest. To enable them to continue to function, this exception allows them to process the data exclusively of their members, provided that such data is not shared outside the organisation without the data subject's consent. Since these organisations work primarily with non-health data, this exemption is not applied to health data to a great extent. On the other hand, the exception that regulates the possibility of processing health data if necessary for establishing, exercising, or defence of legal claims or when courts are acting in their judicial capacity is essential. It is mainly about the victims in cases of injury to health or even death, but also about the possibility of assessing the legal capacity of individual actors.

Letter (j) covers the exception, devoted to research in all areas of importance for society, i.e. not only for public health. Due to the essential ethical and data protection issues of the subject in the research context, the GDPR deals in more detail with the regulation of these rules in Article 89. The application manufacturers may interpret this provision as an opportunity to process the user's health data without their knowledge for their research and benefit. However, it is necessary to observe the rules more closely defined in Article 89 (1), which specifies that without the subject's consent, it is possible to archive and process this data exclusively in the public interest, scientific or historical research purposes or statistical purposes. From this, I believe that if the manufacturers use the user's data for research aimed at profit, this is illegal data processing.

The last exception is only the reformulated recital 52, which I have already mentioned, which allows for reasons of substantial public interest to process data if sufficient guarantees are created at the European or national level to protect the rights of the data subject. This exception is very general and may interfere with the human rights of citizens. Try to imagine it in a situation close to us from past years - the COVID-19 pandemic. Member states have often used this public health exception to protect society against serious cross-border threats. As part of the combination of these exemptions, Member states have started to collect and use citizens' health data to monitor COVID-19 and develop measures to stop the spread of the disease. Health data was thus collected without the citizens' consent, and their other rights, such as the right to freedom of movement or the protection of their privacy, were often affected. On the other hand, exceptions are provided precisely for such binding situations where the individual's right is infringed to protect society. However, this exception contains a clear condition which, in the case of interference with the rights of an individual, must guarantee the protection of their data. The COVID-19 pandemic has shown that using the data available to private companies is possible. On March 22, 2020, Commissioner Thierry Breton summoned all European telephone operators and requested data on the movement of private persons. The operators refused him this data precisely for fear of a violation of the provisions of the GDPR. The Commissar's argument was strictly based on the possibility that "processing is necessary for the performance of the public interest"[38]. If, at that time, health applications were so widespread that they would monitor some critical health information (for example, the temperature) of most of the European population, they would certainly become an interesting target for the EU and individual Member States [32]. Even if this situation is hypothetical, it may occur in the future.

3 The Consent as a Magical Instrument

The last and most used exception in the context of health applications for processing health data is the data subject's consent. Article 9, paragraph 2, letter (a) specifies some consent conditions. It is explicitness for one or more specific purposes. Therefore, it is impossible to grant generic consent without an apparent reason to which it relates. GDPR allows the data subject to give explicit consent for any purpose except where a Member state or the EU provides that the prohibition on processing cannot be lifted by consent. Such cases are sporadic in everyday life. For example, French law provides two cases relating to data concerning the person's health, which must not consider their consent. This is the case of prohibition for the doctor of an insurance company to access a medical file and for an employer to require from a future candidate medical examinations or access to their medical file [17]. However, I am not aware of exceptions that can be connected with health applications.

In addition to these conditions, consent must meet the requirements of Article 7 concerning consent to all personal data. Article 7 describes the principles of the validity of the subject´s consent. The first principle requires that consent must be freely given by the data subject. The second essential principle is that consent must be informed. Although Article 7 does not explicitly use the phrase 'informed consumer', it describes this obligation as making the subject aware of the circumstances of the data processing as well as the possibility of withdrawing the consent given. Article 4 of the GDPR points out in the definition of consent that information is a condition of valid consent:

[...] informed and unambiguous indication of the data subject's wishes by which he or she, by a statement or by a clear affirmative action, signifies agreement to the processing of personal data relating to him or her.

The 'freely given consent' element describes the control the data subject must have over its data. The subject must decide on the consent at any time and, therefore, be able to change or withdraw it. The consent must be considered invalid if it cannot be done without causing detriment. The CJEU, in its decision in the case 'Orange România', also underlined the need for an active role of the data subject linked with the principle of unambiguity of the consent: 'Silence, pre-ticked boxes or inactivity should not, therefore, constitute consent.' [18].

According to the Opinion on Apps on Smart Devices of Article 29 Working Party (WP29), the subject's ability to decide is manifested by control over individual terminations in the data processing framework. This means that it is insufficient for subjects to simply tick the 'Yes, I accept' box if they want to install an application. The application should be able to manage individual data types in detail. According to Article 29 Working Party, such consent is therefore invalid [19]. In reality, this is how most application manufactures behave. Since the CJEU has not yet ruled on the validity of consent in such a situation, it is impossible to support this view with case law. If this were to happen, it would be a breakthrough and an improvement in data protection empowerment for users over their health data in health applications.

When assessing whether consent is freely given, it is necessary to consider the condition under Article 7(4) of GDPR, which does contain a non-exhaustive list of situations when the consent is invalid. It describes that in the case of inappropriate pressure or influence upon the data subject, which prevents a data subject from exercising their free will, it shall render the consent invalid. In principle, this paragraph is aimed especially at situations where a contract is concluded, but not exclusively. As part of the Guidelines 05/2020 on consent under Regulation 2016/679 issued by the European Data Protection Board (EHDB), it provides an example of an application requiring consent for data unrelated to the content provided [21]. If, for example, a step-tracking application provides access to the user's contacts, this request is unauthorised. If it is impossible to use the application without uploading this data, the consent granted for processing it cannot be considered valid. Some health applications tend to have access to the user's contacts, to their other health applications, searches within Internet search engines or even to profiles on social networks. The consent must be considered invalid if the user cannot refuse access to this data separately. The quotation of Opinion, 06/2014 of WP29, underlines the strict character of the interpretation of the necessity to process the data in the link with the concluding contract:

[...] the term "necessary for the performance of a contract" needs to be interpreted strictly. The processing must be necessary to fulfil the contract with each data subject. [21]

If the data processing is not directly connected with the data, the data subject should have a right to deny consent to this operation. Otherwise, the consent in this regard is considered invalid.

The last element associated with free consent is defined by Recital 43 of the GDPR and is often referred to as an 'imbalance of power'. It focuses on the unequal position between the data subject and the controller, especially about the public authority or employer. Due to the existing dominance of the controller, it is necessary to guarantee the data is subject to greater protection against emerging pressure. Again, the principle applies that consent is considered invalid if it is impossible to express consent to all types of data separately and, therefore, not allow access to some personal data. Even if it can be argued that this provision does not concern health applications, the EHDB points out that imbalances of power are not limited to public authorities and employers; they may also occur in other situations [21]. It points to the opinion of WP29 that if the data subject is not able to exercise a real choice without the risk of deception, intimidation, coercion, or significant negative consequences, then the consent is always invalid [36]. Especially considering health applications focused on mental health, the imbalance of power can be significant. There is noticeable pressure because the users often need urgent help, which they do not receive regularly. Thus, they agree to all the conditions for the sole purpose of downloading the application and getting help. Based on a study that examined user reviews of mental health applications, users complain about non-transparency. Users criticise that they download an application when already feeling low, just to realise that the support they need is available only under other conditions, where one shares data unrelated to the application. Due to their urgent need to solve their health problems, the manufacturers exploit their vulnerabilities, and their consent is invalid [23].

On the other hand, researchers point out that fulfilling the principles set out in recitals 42 and 43 concerning power imbalances is burdensome and difficult to achieve, if possible, in the health field [24]. Based on the example of an imbalance of power given by the EDPB, for example, a situation where a patient:

[...] is not in good health conditions when participants belong to an economically or socially disadvantaged group or in any institutional or hierarchical dependency situation. [26]

Since the users of these applications are often vulnerable and decide on the most precious thing, their health, it is difficult to find this balance. In conclusion, I state the necessity to approach this problem more sensitively regarding health data.

The second element is granting consent for one or more specific purposes as set out in Article 9(2)(a). The so-called granularity of consent is vital. This means that in the case of data processing for several purposes, the subject must consent to each purpose separately and independently. Thus, the subject can decide to give consent to the processing of data for their use of the health application (their own benefit) but can refuse to allow the data to be used for statistical or advertising purposes.

Closely linked to this element is the possibility of the subject withdrawing consent at any time for any purpose. An essential condition in Article 7(3) of GDPR stipulates that withdrawing consent must be as simple as giving it. However, for health applications, this condition is challenging to meet, especially because consent is usually confirmed with a one-mouse click. As I have mentioned above, this is already contrary to the granting of valid consent since it must be granted separately for each purpose. The same should be the case if the subject wants to withdraw consent. For this reason, health applications should allow users to access and withdraw their consent at any time with a few clicks. A particular case is set when the application uses access to another application within the mobile device, for example, for location measurement. The subject has the right to withdraw consent for location measurement. If, based on this withdrawal of consent, the application ceases to function, there is a breach of recital 42 under the EHDB. More precisely, a detriment to the data subject is created, and the consent is therefore invalid from the outset [21]. The controller must destroy all the data obtained while using the application. This interpretation is essential for health applications that often use other devices or applications to collect data to evaluate the subject's health status.

The last element is the informed subject because only a subject with objective information regarding personal data processing can provide informed consent. Although GDPR does not define how informed consent should look like, the General Advocate's interpretation of the case 'Orange România' lists the data that the subject must know to give informed consent:

In particular, [data subject] must know which data are to be processed, the duration of such processing, in what way and for which specific purpose. [...] who is processing the data and whether the data are intended to be transferred to third parties. [data subject] must be informed of the consequences of refusing consent... [39]

The CJEU decision confirms the Advocate General's opinion and adds that the controller should also inform whether the answers to the questions are mandatory or voluntary and what the possible consequences are of not answering. The health applications usually contain all this information in the section appearing immediately after downloading the application - 'terms and conditions'. Most of the time, the users will only see a checkbox that asks them to approve a sentence that confirms the terms and conditions. Of course, it is possible to read them if the user wants. However a study from 2017 shows that 91% of users do not read the terms of use and only confirm that they have read them before installing the app. This can be considered as the user´s negligence [27]. GDPR provides sufficient protection, but if the users do not exercise their rights, it is impossible to protect their personal data to the full extent, i.e., it is the user's fault. However, it is crucial to think about this user´s behaviour. Research shows that users of apps emphasise that it does not matter whether they read the terms and conditions or not if they need the application [25]. If they disagree with the terms and conditions, they cannot use the health application and get the treatment they expect. In the section mentioned above, this consent is invalid. The solution to this problem is to meet the granularity of consent. If the user could refuse certain types of data processing independent of the ability to use the app, 67% of users would click and read the terms and conditions. This data shows that almost two-thirds of users would increase the protection of their personal data if the manufacturers of health applications respected the requirements for consent [27].

Users have also identified another reason for not reading the terms of apps: their complexity and the use of legal or technical language that is not understandable. Recital 42 specifies the wording of the consent if it is predefined by the controller (in this case, the manufacturer of the application): '[consent] should be provided in an intelligible and easily accessible form, using clear and plain language and it should not contain the unfair term.' [25].

WP29 specifies that in the case of the use of overly complicated legal or too technical jargon, the consent is invalid. Thus, if the conditions of application frequently refer to legislation without explaining the principle itself, the consent is invalid. This is directly related to the WP29 condition that the language must be suitable for the subject, i.e., suitability is judged by the subject's ability to understand the conditions [40]. Unfortunately, I cannot but conclude that many health applications use it as a standard practice not to observe this condition of consent. The user often does not want to go into dispute with the manufacturer. Neither the EU nor the Member states can control the conformity of all applications with GDPR. For this reason, manufacturers often abuse their position vis-à-vis users to benefit from their data, which are a valuable commodity to trade.

All the conditions mentioned above are necessary elements of valid consent of the data subject for proceeding with their personal health data. Subject consent is the most common, and in the case of health applications, almost unique way of legally processing the subject's health data. Based on these practices, the health data is still processed even if valid consent is not provided.

4 Conclusion

In conclusion, this article undertook a comprehensive exploration of the intricate landscape surrounding the utilisation of health data within health applications. Through a focused analysis, I sought to unravel the critical considerations entailed in processing such data while operating within the framework of health applications. The inquiry extended beyond the mere purview of legal provisions, encompassing a holistic examination of judicial precedents and authoritative recommendations that dictate the acquisition of user consent for health data processing. The discernment gleaned from the Court of Justice of the European Union's verdict notably underscores the well-defined contours of consent principles within the realm of health data.

However, the seamless translation of these principles into the practical realm of health applications remains deficient. The prevalent deficiencies inherent in health applications often engender inadequacies that compromise the freedom of users' consent. A salient instance lies in the prevalent practice of procuring consent through a single click, for countless purpose under the umbrella of "terms and conditions." This methodological approach starkly deviates from the foundational doctrine of granular consent, thus curtailing users' to selectively endorse specific purposes of these provisions. Consequently, the ability to withhold consent for the collection of users' health-related data via application usage is considerably diminished. This phenomenon frequently extends to scenarios where user data might be repurposed for unrelated objectives, such as advertising or research endeavors that diverge from the core health application functionality. Moreover, this imbalance of power between application manufacturers and users becomes particularly pronounced, as users are often coerced into compliance due to the importance of the application for their health, even if their personal convictions diverge.

In light of these predicaments, it is crucial to acknowledge that although extant legal frameworks and judicial interpretations furnish safeguards against data breaches and unauthorised data utilisation, the existing shortcomings primarily manifest in invalidity of the user's consent. The predicament is not solely confined to data leakage but pertains to the improper manipulation of user data. Examples abound where health applications accumulate data surpassing operational necessity or given the unbalance of power, pressure users to give up data that predominantly serves the financial interests of the application manufacturers rather than serving the application functionalities.

Consequently, while the legal and jurisprudential foundation upholds user health data protection, the efficacy thereof is tempered by the lack of robust controlling mechanisms and the practical constraints associated with overseeing the multitude of approximately 370,000 health applications. Nevertheless, avenues for fortification persist.

Foremost among these is the imperative to empower users with an comprehension of their rights, to promote awareness regarding the need for informed consent. Additionally, fostering the dissemination and implementation of best practices within the manufacturer community—ranging from facilitating consent withdrawal mechanisms, to transparent notifications concerning changes in data processing—holds the potential to yield progression. The combination of these two essential elements, encompassing user education and manufacturer best practices, is promising to creat an ecosystem wherein the of user's health data finds enhanced safeguarding.

References

1. Buchholz, K.: Where Health App Usage Is Most Common. https://www.statista.com/chart/23161/health-app-usage-country-comparison/. Accessed 8 Aug 2023
2. SMER: The Quantified Human. Ethical aspects on self monitoring by wearables and health apps. https://smer.se/. Accessed 15 Aug 2023
3. Eurostat: Aging Europe - Statistics on Population Developments. https://ec.europa.eu/eurostat/statistics-explained/index.php?title=Ageing_Europe_-_statistics_on_population_developments#Older_people_.E2.80.94_population_overview. Accessed 23 Aug 2023
4. Eurostat: Mental Health and Related Issues Statistics. https://ec.europa.eu/eurostat/statistics-explained/index.php?title=Mental_health_and_related_issues_statistics#Extent_of_depressive_disorders. Accessed 14 Aug 2023
5. European Commission: Green Paper on Mobile Health. https://digital-strategy.ec.europa.eu/en/library/green-paper-mobile-health-mhealth. Accessed 29 Aug 2023
6. Kleinman, Z.: Most Healthcare Apps not up to NHS Standards. https://www.bbc.com/news/technology-56083231.amp. Accessed 29 Aug 2023
7. IQVIA: Digital Health Trends 2021. https://cens.cl/wp-content/uploads/2022/02/Biblio-iqvia-institute-digital-health-trends-2021.pdf. Accessed 29 Aug 2023

8. ORCHA: The Peoples´ View of Digital Mental Health. https://25077478.fs1.hubspotus ercontent-eu1.net/hubfs/25077478/Mental%20health%20campaign/Digital%20for%20M ental%20Health%20Attitudes%20and%20Behaviour%20Report.pdf?__hstc=14005480.6b5 6432c0c0d0df557f77e3260f80339.1675850072907.1676295687602.1676747717589.6&__ hssc=14005480.3.1676747717589&__hsfp=2806405925. Accessed 29 Aug 2023
9. E-hälsomyndigheten: Hälsoappar Södertätt och Ubandärung. https://www.ehalsomyndig heten.se/globalassets/ehm/3_om-oss/rapporter/halsoappar---forutsattningar-och-anvand ning.pdf. Accessed 29 Aug 2023
10. ORCHA: Digital & Mental Health Recovery Actions Plans. https://orchahealth.com/wp-con tent/uploads/2021/04/Mental_Health_Report_2021_final.pdf. Accessed 29 Aug 2023
11. Case C-219/115 Brain Products GmbH v BioSemi VOF e.a [2012] ECJ 2012/11
12. Batya Swift, Y.: An Uncomfortable Truth: Why Patients Lie to Their Physicians. https:// www.empr.com/home/features/an-uncomfortable-truth-why-patients-lie-to-their-physic ians/. Accessed 15 Aug 2023
13. Sawrikar, V., Mote, K.: Technology acceptance and trust: Overlooked considerations in young people's use of digital mental health interventions. Health Policy and Technol. **11**(4) (2022)
14. Lustgarten, S., Garrison, Y., Sinnard, M., Flynn, A.: Digital privacy in mental healthcare: current issues and recommendations for technology use. Curr. Opin. Psychol. **36**, 25–31 (2020)
15. Kretzschmar, K., Tyroll, H., Pavarini, G., Manzini, A., Singh, I.: Can your phone be your therapist? young people's ethical perspectives on the use of fully automated conversational agents (Chatbots) in mental health support. Biomedical Informatics Insights **11** (2019)
16. Maaß, L., et al.: The definitions of health apps and medical apps from the perspective of public health and law: qualitative analysis of an interdisciplinary literature overview. JMIR Mhealth Uhealth **10** (2022)
17. Bossi, J.: Technologies de l'information et de la communication et donnees de sante : pour un cadre juridique en phase avec les évolutions technologiques et les besoins du systeme de sante. Statistique et Société **2**(33)
18. C-61/19 Orange Romania SA v Autoritatea Națională de Supraveghere a Prelucrării Datelor cu Caracter Personal [2020] ERC 2020/901
19. Article 29 Working Party: Opinion on Apps on Mobile Devices. https://ec.europa.eu/jus tice/article-29/documentation/opinion-recommendation/files/2013/wp202_en.pdf. Accessed 16 Aug 2023
20. World Health Organization: Ethics and Governance of Artificial Intelligence for Health. https://www.who.int/publications/i/item/9789240029200. Accessed 6 Aug 2023
21. European Data Protection Board: Guidelines 05/2020 on Consent under Regulation 2016/679. https://edpb.europa.eu/sites/default/files/files/file1/edpb_guidelines_202005_con sent_en.pdf. Accessed 26 Aug 2023
22. Batya Swift, Y.: An Uncomfortable Truth: Why Patients Lie to Their Physicians. http:// www.empr.com/home/features/an-uncomfortable-truth-why-patients-lie-to-their-physic ians/. Accessed 21 Aug 2023
23. Haque, R., Rubya, S.: For an app supposed to make its users feel better, it sure is a joke" - an analysis of user reviews of mobile mental health applications. 6 Proceedings of the ACM Conference on Human-Computer Interaction **6**(2), 1–29 (2022)
24. Kirwan, M., et al.: What GDPR and the health research regulations (HRRs) mean for Ireland: "explicit consent"—a legal analysis. Ir J. Med. Sci. **515**(190) (2021)
25. Liu, Y.: User control of personal information concerning mobile app: notice and consent? Computer Law & Security Review **30**(5) (2014)

26. European Data Protection Board: Opinion 3/2019 concerning the Questions and Answers on the Interplay Between the Clinical Trials Regulation (CTR) and the General Data Protection Regulation. https://edpb.europa.eu/sites/default/files/files/file1/edpb_opinionctrq_a_final_en.pdf. Accessed 19 Aug 2023
27. Deloitte: Global Mobile Consumer Survey: US edition. https://www2.deloitte.com/content/dam/Deloitte/us/Documents/technology-media-telecommunications/us-tmt-2017-global-mobile-consumer-survey-executive-summary.pdf. Accessed 19 Aug 2023
28. European Commission, Proposal for a Regulation of the European Parliament and of the Council laying down harmonised rules on Artificial intelligence and amending certain union legislative acts. COM/2021/206 final
29. Keskinbora, K.H.: Medical ethics considerations on artificial intelligence. J. Clin. Neurosci. **64**, 277–282 (2019)
30. Andorno, R.: The Oviedo convention: a European legal framework at the intersection of human rights and health law. J. Int. Biotechnol. Law **2**(4), 133–143 (2005)
31. Charter of Fundamental Rights of the European Union, C 326/391. http://data.europa.eu/eli/reg/2017/745/oj
32. Hossfeld, C.H., Muller-Lagarde, Y., Alexander, D., Pöschke, M., Zevounou, L.: European Public Interest. https://hal.science/hal-01936960/document. Accessed 19 July 2023
33. Regulation (EU) 2016/679. The protection of natural persons with regard to the processing of personal data and on the free movement of such data. European Parliament and Council. http://data.europa.eu/eli/reg/2016/679/oj
34. Regulation (EC) No 1338/2008 of the European Parliament and of the Council of 16 December 2008 on Community statistics on public health and health and safety at work. http://data.europa.eu/eli/reg/2008/1338/oj
35. Regulation (EU) 2017/745 of the European Parliament and of the Council of 5 April 2017 on medical devices, amending Directive 2001/83/EC, Regulation (EC) No 178/2002 and Regulation (EC) No 1223/2009 and repealing Council Directives 90/385/EEC and 93/42/EEC. European Parliament and Council. http://data.europa.eu/eli/reg/2017/745/oj
36. Article 29 Working Party: Opinion 15/2011 on the definition of consent. https://ec.europa.eu/justice/article-29/documentation/opinion-recommendation/files/2011/wp187_en.pdf. Accessed 10 Oct 2023
37. Directive 95/46/EC of the European Parliament and of the Council of 24 October 1995 on the protection of individuals with regard to the processing of personal data and on the free movement of such data. http://data.europa.eu/eli/dir/1995/46/oj
38. Politico: Commission tells carriers to hand over mobile data in coronavirus fight. https://www.politico.eu/article/european-commission-mobile-phone-data-thierry-breton-coronavirus-covid19/. Accessed 2 Oct 2024
39. Opinion of Advocate General Szpunar, Case C-61/19, Orange Romania SA v Autoritatea Nationala de Supraveghere a Prelucrarii Datelor cu Caracter Personal (2020).
40. Article 29 Working Party: Guidelines on transparency under Regulation 2016/679. https://ec.europa.eu/newsroom/article29/redirection/document/51025. Accessed 1 Oct 2024

The Application of Virtual Reality in Enhancing Medical Education: Benefits, Challenges, and Outlook for the Future

Seydou Golo Barro[1,2,3], Delwêndé Serge Lebian Wilfried Nikiema[1,2,4(✉)], Yves Kantagba[1,2], and Pascal Staccini[3]

[1] Université Nazi BONI de Bobo Dioulasso, Bobo Dioulasso, Burkina Faso
[2] Centre de Formation et de Recherche en Technologies Médicales (CFRTM), Bobo Dioulasso, Burkina Faso
[3] RETINES - Université Côte d'Azur, Nice, France
[4] Burkina Institute of Technology(BIT), Koudougou, Burkina Faso
lebian.nikiema@bit.bf

Abstract. This article discusses the revolution of medical education through immersive learning experiences in Virtual Reality (VR). It highlights the advantages, challenges, and future advancements of VR in medical education. The benefits of VR include immersive and interactive scenarios that help students understand complex medical concepts and empower personalized and self-directed learning. However, implementing VR in medical education is difficult due to technical challenges and potential physiological side effects. Despite these challenges, the growth of the VR industry offers hope for transforming medical education by closing gaps, increasing accessibility, and encouraging collaboration. The article emphasizes the need for collaboration among educators, researchers, and institutions to fully harness the transformative potential of VR in medical education. It concludes by stating that VR not only transforms medical education technologically but also changes how medical knowledge is acquired, internalized, and applied, creating a dynamic and immersive learning experience for future healthcare professionals.

Keywords: Virtual reality · Medical education · Immersive learning · Simulation-based training · Pedagogical innovation · VR applications

1 Introduction

The current state of medical education is confronted with ever-changing challenges, which in turn drive the development of technological advancements aimed at enhancing the quality of learning experiences. Conventional methodologies frequently encounter challenges in effectively captivating contemporary learners.

As a response, educators are currently investigating novel methodologies that utilize technology to establish connections between theoretical knowledge and practical skills. Among these technological advancements, Virtual Reality (VR) is identified as a powerful tool for transforming medical education. This article delves into the various implications of incorporating virtual reality (VR) into medical education, providing insight into its advantages, obstacles, and potential avenues for future development.

2 Definition and Basics of Virtual Reality

Virtual Reality (VR) is a complicated mix of philosophy and technology. Its definition has expanded to include several aspects, making it multidimensional [19]. The 18th-century philosophy of Immanuel Kant inspired VR's creation. Kant's philosophy distinguished subjective mental experiences from objective external facts [13]. Modern "Virtual Reality" refers to a computer-mediated interface that enhances immersion, realism, and interactivity in a digital world [11]. Jaron Lanier popularized this interface, which combines computer science with behavioral interfaces for instant virtual interactions [6].

VR is based on "3I"-immersion, interaction, and imagination [3]. Immersion blurs the line between reality and virtuality via sensory reactions. Interaction allows users to actively shape and change the virtual environment, improving learning engagement and ownership. VR relies on imagination to suspend disbelief and enhance realism. In the 1990s, virtual presence changed from coexisting with others. It included participants' subjective sensations, producing a deep feeling of "being there" [19]. Immersion is like sinking into water, suggesting willingness to respond with compelling stimuli [15]. Education nowadays relies on tactile and digital immersion. Simulations, role plays, and games encourage active participation [16]. VR, AR, and MR provide dynamic instructional environments [18]. Immersive technologies and instructional methods interact dynamically in experiential education.

3 Virtual Reality Applications in Medical Education

The introduction of Virtual Reality (VR) technology into medical education has resulted in significant changes, effectively tackling important issues like the retention of knowledge and the smooth integration of theoretical concepts with practical applications [7]. Traditional approaches to communicating intricate medical concepts have frequently proven inadequate in satisfying the requirements of modern education. Nevertheless, the implementation of virtual reality (VR) technology has surfaced as a proficient approach, specifically for senior surgical residents who reap advantages from its ability to offer immediate feedback and foster active learning [7]. The worldwide transition to online education, accelerated by the COVID-19 pandemic, has additionally emphasized the significance of virtual reality (VR) in clinical teaching [7]. Scientists in the respective domain highly praise virtual reality (VR) as a training technique owing to its capacity to augment comprehension and the acquisition of skills, notwithstanding potential financial considerations [7]. The integration of virtual reality (VR) technology with conventional teaching methods, particularly in undergraduate medical education, is a rapidly growing phenomenon that is expected to bring about substantial transformations in the field of medical learning [7]. The continuous investigation into the effects of virtual reality immersion on learning outcomes, habits, performance, and graduation rates in the field of medical education continues to be an important research pursuit [7]. The applications of virtual reality have a substantial reach in the field of medical anatomy education [12]. This novel technology provides a viable alternative to traditional two-dimensional illustrations by allowing students to actively interact with intricate anatomical structures of the human body in real-time. The immersive learning experience is enhanced by the creation of virtual humans, which are sophisticated digital replicas that incorporate human biology, morphology, and physics to facilitate scientific investigation [10]. In the field of surgical education, the incorporation of Virtual Surgery Simulation Systems (VSSS) surpasses the conventional practices of utilizing cadavers and anthropometric dummies [12]. This transition facilitates surgical trainees with a platform for practical implementation, augmenting psychomotor abilities, coordination, and ambidextrous surgical proficiencies [1]. Empirical evidence substantiates the superiority of simulation-based training in relation to performance outcomes when compared to non-simulation-based methodologies [1]. VR applications enhance surgeon confidence and situational awareness by promoting gradual skill improvement in a controlled setting that allows for errors [1]. The cumulative effect of these applications fundamentally transforms pedagogical methodologies, creating opportunities for skilled healthcare practitioners [1].

4 Benefits of Virtual Reality in Medical Education

The integration of virtual reality simulations represents a significant shift in the field, posing a challenge to traditional approaches that heavily depend on the use of cadavers and animals [22]. Virtual reality (VR) technology has been found to provide unique benefits for clinical skills training. One such advantage is the creation of safe and customized learning environments that promote self-directed and personalized learning experiences [24]. The traditional methodology of "observe one, perform one, instruct one" in surgical education is currently facing reduced acceptance as a result of apprehensions regarding patient safety and the financial consequences of medical errors on healthcare institutions [19]. The user's text is already scientific. The advantages of virtual reality (VR) encompass a wide range of recipients, such as individuals engaged in the process of acquiring knowledge, academic staff, and the entirety of the healthcare system. The system enhances the efficiency of accessing clinical experiences, effectively incorporates simulation-based education into real-world applications, and maximizes the improvement of skills. The replicability of virtual reality (VR) simulations and the psychological security they provide present an attractive alternative to conventional simulation centers, effectively addressing constraints on resources [17]. Furthermore, virtual reality (VR) programs effectively involve learners, promoting the development of cognitive, psychomotor, and communication abilities, placing learners at the core of the learning process [10].

5 Challenges and Limitations of VR in Medical Education

Although virtual reality (VR) exhibits significant potential, it also poses various obstacles. One notable challenge that arises is the possibility of cybersickness, which encompasses a range of symptoms such as nausea, vertigo, and ocular discomfort that are encountered by certain users [19]. The educational potential of virtual reality (VR) is accompanied by apprehensions regarding quality assurance. The presence of variability in software specifications and the contrasting nature of diverse research and development (R&D) standards among companies requires educators to thoroughly assess different options in order to attain the most favorable teaching outcomes [24]. Continuing scientific investigation is currently examining the immediate impacts of virtual reality (VR) on the visual attention and ocular alignment. The intricate relationship between accommodation (the adjustment of the eyes' focus) and convergence (the alignment of the eyes to focus on a single point) renders these ocular effects notably intricate, particularly when employing head-mounted displays [4].

6 Pedagogical Aspects of Virtual Reality

The transformative potential of virtual reality (VR) extends beyond its mere technological novelty. It facilitates a significant transformation in pedagogical methodologies within the field of medical education. In accordance with rigorous pedagogical standards, virtual reality (VR) effectively combines various components such as hardware, software, and procedural complexities to generate fully engaging educational settings [9]. The constructivist theory of learning has gained prominence in recent years, highlighting the importance of experiential learning as a complement to traditional approaches [5]. The versatility of virtual reality (VR) is clearly demonstrated in its applications in nursing, patient simulation, and surgical practice, leading to a transformative impact on education within the healthcare field [2]. By engaging learners in active participation, virtual reality (VR) technology improves cognitive, psychomotor, and communication skills [10]. The integration of theoretical knowledge and practical application through immersive, experiential learning journeys has a transformative effect on medical education, cultivating a future cohort of proficient healthcare professionals [2].

7 Case Study and Examples

Institutions worldwide are utilizing virtual reality (VR) technology to enhance medical education. An exemplary instance can be observed in the collaboration between Taipei Medical University and HTC, which led to the development of the largest virtual reality (VR) anatomy class in the world [21]. This novel solution offers access to a collection of more than 4,000 intricate 3D anatomical models, accommodating the requirements of up to 300 online students concurrently. The utilization of virtual reality technology in this approach enhances students' understanding of anatomy and provides them with a thorough knowledge base for specialized areas within the medical field [21] (Fig. 1). The University of Northampton and the University of Oxford are leading institutions in the integration of virtual reality (VR) technology into medical education. The primary objectives of their endeavors revolve around providing instruction to healthcare practitioners, nursing students, and physicians within a virtual reality (VR) setting that is both conducive and secure [14]. These case studies highlight the tangible effects of virtual reality (VR) in the field of medical education, surpassing conventional teaching methods and facilitating engaging and immersive learning opportunities [24].

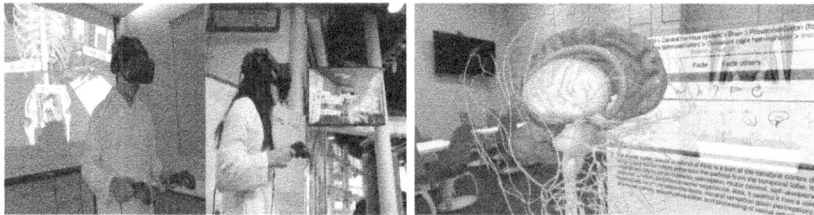

Fig. 1. Taipei University students in practice in Anatomy 3D Simulator

8 Future Trends and Directions

Virtual Reality (VR) is currently transforming the landscape of medical education through the implementation of several cutting-edge advancements. These include the utilization of medical simulations, integration of haptic feedback, incorporation of adaptive learning algorithms, enhancement of mobile VR accessibility, and the establishment of community VR platforms. These technological advancements are enhancing the educational experience for medical students by facilitating improved training methods and enhancing their comprehension of intricate medical concepts. These immersive environments facilitate the preparation of real-life scenarios, the development of devices, the study of treatment and therapy, and the advancement of medical research in the field of driving [23]. The integration of haptic feedback enhances the authenticity and immersion of learning environments, while adaptive learning algorithms employ data analytics to personalize learning journeys according to individual progress. The utilization of portable devices in mobile virtual reality (VR) enhances the accessibility and flexibility of VR education. This allows for on-the-go learning and promotes a culture of continuous medical education. Community VR is a ground-breaking technology that transforms the way collaborative learning occurs, allowing learners to establish connections and engage with one another in virtual environments. This innovation has a profound impact on medical education, as it significantly enhances engagement and promotes collaboration among students. In general, virtual reality (VR) has the potential to significantly impact the medical education domain, fundamentally altering the methods through which medical professionals receive training and education [8]. The estimated valuation of the VR and Augmented Reality (AR) sector reaching $35 billion by 2025 highlights its significant growth prospects [20] (Fig. 2). As the field progresses, the applications of virtual reality (VR) are poised to have a significant impact on the realm of medical education and practice. This calls for an active and forward-thinking strategy towards conducting research, fostering innovation, and promoting collaboration in order to effectively leverage the transformative capabilities of virtual reality (VR).

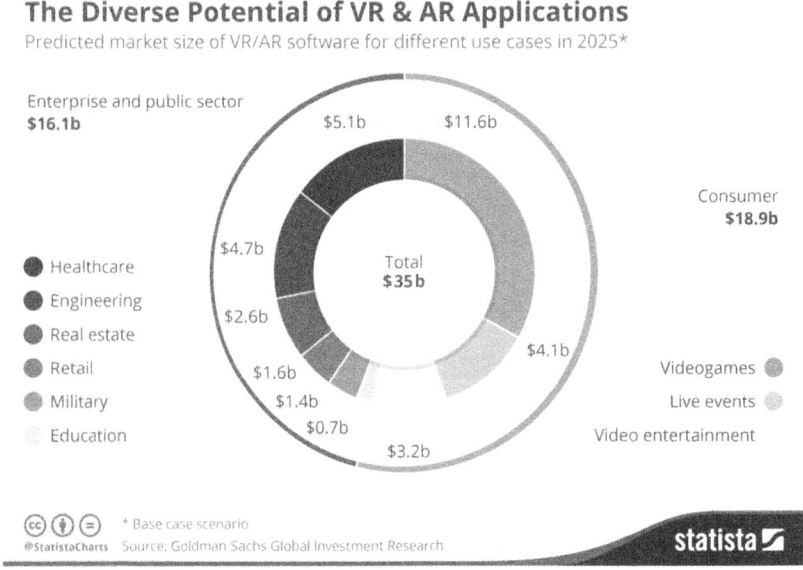

Fig. 2. Statista trends and predictions about VR/AR market in 2025

9 Conclusion

VR is transforming medical education through immersive and interactive learning. It enhances psychomotor abilities and situational awareness by letting students engage with complex anatomical components in real time, bypassing traditional instructional methods. VR applications provide novel nursing, patient simulation, dental training, and surgical practice. However, discomfort, cybersickness, and quality requirements across multiple software specifications make VR incorporation in medical education difficult. Despite these obstacles, VR in medical education will alter the field. Medical simulations in VR will improve training, haptic feedback technology will add a tactile element, adaptive learning algorithms will customize instruction, and mobile VR will democratize immersive education. For team-based medical education, community VR platforms encourage cooperation and shared learning. The VR market is anticipated to reach $80 billion by 2025, transforming medical education. To maximize its potential, educators, researchers, and healthcare organizations must innovate and collaborate. To use VR's revolutionary power, research, investment, and curriculum creation must be proactive. The revolutionary impact of VR will help future healthcare workers understand its intricacies.

References

1. Agha, R.A., Fowler, A.J.: The role and validity of surgical simulation. Int. Surg. **100**(2), 350–357 (2015). https://doi.org/10.9738/INTSURG-D-14-00004.1
2. Asad, M.M., Naz, A., Churi, P., Tahanzadeh, M.M.: Virtual reality as pedagogical tool to enhance experiential learning: a systematic literature review. Educ. Res. Int. **2021**, 1–17 (2021). Hindawi Limited
3. Bamodu, O., Ye, X.M.: Virtual reality and virtual reality system components. Adv. Mater. Res. **765–767**, 1169–1172 (2013). https://doi.org/10.4028/www.scientific.net/AMR.765-767.1169
4. Che Azemin, M.Z.: Short term effect of virtual reality on eye accommodative ability. J. Eng. Sci. Res. **4**(1), 35–39 (2020). RMP Publications
5. Fallman, D., Backman, A., Holmlund, K.: VR in education: an introduction to multisensory constructivist learning environments (2013). https://urn.kb.se/resolve?urn=urn:nbn:se:umu:diva-81668
6. Fuchs, P.G.M., Stéphane, D.: Le traité de la réalité virtuelle. Presses des MINES, 2nd edn (2009)
7. Gan, W., et al.: Researching the application of virtual reality in medical education: one-year follow-up of a randomized trial. BMC Med. Educ. **23**(1) (2023). Springer Science and Business Media LLC
8. ixrlabs. Top Technological Trends and Virtual Reality for Medical Education. https://www.ixrlabs.com/blog/top-technological-trends-and-virtual-reality-for-medical-education/
9. Johnston, E., Olivas, G., Steele, P., Smith, C., Bailey, L.: Exploring pedagogical foundations of existing virtual reality educational applications: a content analysis study. J. Educ. Technol. Syst. **46**(4), 414–439 (2017). SAGE Publications
10. Kim, Y.Y., Kim, E.N., Park, M.J., Park, K.S., Ko, H.D., Kim, H.T.: The application of biosignal feedback for reducing cybersickness from exposure to a virtual environment. Presence: Teleoper. Virt. Environ. **17**(1), 1–16 (2008). MIT Press - Journals
11. Krueger, M.W.: An easy entry artificial reality. In: Virtual Reality, pp. 147–161 (1993). Elsevier
12. Lai, P., Zou, W.: The application of virtual reality technology in medical education and training. Glob. J. Inf. Technol. Emerg. Technol. **8**(1), 10–15 (2018). Birlesik Dunya Yenilik Arastirma ve Yayincilik Merkezi

13. LaValle, S.M.: Virtual Reality. Cambridge University Press (2023)
14. Mergen, M., Meyerheim, M., Graf, N.: Reviewing the current state of virtual reality integration in medical education - a scoping review protocol. Syst. Rev. **12**(1) (2023). Springer Science and Business Media LLC
15. Mystakidis, S., Lympouridis, V.: Immersive learning. Encyclopedia **3**(2), 396–405 (2023). MDPI AG
16. Nygaard, C., Courtney, N., Leigh, E.: Simulations, Games and Role Play in University Education, vol. 1-22. Libri Publishing, Faringdon (2012)
17. Pottle, J.: Virtual reality and the transformation of medical education. Future Healthc. J. **6**(3), 181–185 (2019). Royal College of Physicians
18. Rauschnabel, P.A., Felix, R., Hinsch, C., Shahab, H., Alt, F.: What is XR? Towards a framework for augmented and virtual reality. Comput. Hum. Behav. **133**, 107289 (2022). Elsevier BV
19. Riener, R., Harders, M.: Introduction to virtual reality in medicine. In: Riener, R., Harders, M. (eds.) Virtual Reality in Medicine, pp. 1–12. Springer, London (2012). https://doi.org/10.1007/978-1-4471-4011-5_1
20. Sik-Lanyi, C.: Virtual reality healthcare system could be a potential future of health consultations. In: 2017 IEEE 30th Neumann Colloquium (NC). IEEE (2017)
21. University, T.M.: TMU pioneers world's largest virtual reality anatomy class - Office of Global Engagement (2019). https://oge.tmu.edu.tw/tmu-pioneers-worlds-largest-virtual-reality-anatomy-class-2/
22. Ustun, A.B., Yilmaz, R., Karaoglan Yilmaz, F.G.: Virtual reality in medical education. In: Advances in Medical Technologies and Clinical Practice, pp. 56–73. IGI Global (2020)
23. VR, M.: How VR is Changing the Future of Medical Education (2023). https://www.linkedin.com/pulse/how-vr-changing-future-medical-education-medisim-vr
24. Yu, W., Wen, L., Zhao, L.A., Liu, X., Wang, B., Yang, H.: The applications of virtual reality technology in medical education: a review and mini-research. J. Phys.: Conf. Ser. **1176**, 022055 (2019). IOP Publishing

Author Index

A
Ahad, Abdul 14, 44
Ali, Zahra 44
Almeida, Edwing A. 57
Asadipour, Ali 65
Ashfaq, Fiza 14

B
Barro, Seydou Golo 131
Berry, Damon 33
Bhatt, Kavita 84
Buitrón, Marcela E. 57

D
Doyle, Julie 33

H
Hussain, Mudassar 14

K
Kantagba, Yves 131
Karman, Ian 97
Kumar, S. Mohan 84

M
Madeira, Filipe 14, 44
Marron, Ann 33
Martínez, Julieta 57
Mazur-Milecka, Magdalena 3
Miranda, Jorge 3

Mohsenvand, Mostafa 'Neo' 97
Müllerová, Petra 117

N
Nikiema, Delwêndé Serge Lebian Wilfried 131
Nugent, Ciarán 33

O
O'Sullivan, Dympna 33

P
Pourshahrokhi, Narges 65

R
Rumiński, Jacek 3

S
Shayea, Ibraheem 44
Silva, Jose A. 97
Soroushmojdehi, Rahil 97
Staccini, Pascal 131
Sun, Yitong 65
Sun, Yue 97

T
Turner, Jonathan 33

W
Wagner, Stefan Rahr 3
Wilson, Michael 33

SPRINGER NATURE

GPSR Compliance

The European Union's (EU) General Product Safety Regulation (GPSR) is a set of rules that requires consumer products to be safe and our obligations to ensure this.

If you have any concerns about our products, you can contact us on ProductSafety@springernature.com

In case Publisher is established outside the EU, the EU authorized representative is:

Springer Nature Customer Service Center GmbH
Europaplatz 3
69115 Heidelberg, Germany

The manufacturer's authorised representative in the EU is Springer Nature Customer Service Centre GmbH, Europaplatz 3, 69115 Heidelberg, Germany. If you have any concerns regarding our products, please contact ProductSafety@springernature.com

Printed and bound by CPI Group (UK) Ltd, Croydon, CR0 4YY

25/03/2026

02078190-0013